MULTIPLE OBJECTIVE TREATMENT ASPECTS OF BANK FILTRATION

Multiple Objective Treatment Aspects of Bank Filtration

DISSERTATION

by

Submitted in fulfillment of the requirements of
the Board for Doctorates of Delft University of Technology
and of the Academic Board of the UNESCO-IHE Institute for Water Education for the
Degree of DOCTOR
to be defended in public
on Friday, October 29, 2010 at 10:00 hours
in Delft, the Netherlands
Sung Kyu Maeng
born in Seoul , South Korea

Master of Science in Environmental Engineering
Georgia Institute of Science and Technology, USA

This dissertation has been approved by the supervisor
Prof. dr. G.L. Amy

Members of Awarding Committee;

Chairman	Rector Magnificus, TU Delft, the Netherlands
Vice-chairman	Prof. dr. A. Szöllösi-Nagy, UNESCO-IHE, the Netherlands
Prof. dr. G.L. Amy	UNESCO-IHE, the Netherlands, promotor
Prof. dr. J.C. van Dijk	TU Delft, the Netherlands, copromotor
Dr. S.K. Sharma	UNESCO-IHE, the Netherlands
Prof. dr. T. Grischek	University of Applied Sciences Dresden, Germany
Prof. dr. C. Ray	University of Hawaii at Manoa, USA
Dr. K-H. Ahn	Korea Institute of Science and Technology, South Korea
Prof. dr. D. Brdjanovic	TU Delft, the Netherlands, reserve

CRC Press/Balkema is an imprint of the Taylor & Francis Group, an informa business

Published by:
CRC Press/Balkema
PO Box 447, 2300 AK Leiden, The Netherlands
e-mail: Pub.NL@taylorandfrancis.com
www.crcpress.com – www.taylorandfrancis.co.uk – www.balkema.nl

ISBN 978-0-415-61577-8 (Taylor & Francis Group)

Abstract

The need for safe and good quality drinking water is growing rapidly worldwide, especially with increased urbanization and population growth. However, increasing pollution of surface waters, often by wastewater effluents, has made water treatment more difficult and expensive. Furthermore, most water resources, especially surface waters in industrialized and urban areas in developing countries, are quickly deteriorating as a result of uncontrolled waste discharges into receiving waters, which may also serve as drinking water sources. Consequently, this has led to the occurrence of potentially harmful organic micropollutants (OMPs) in drinking water treatment systems and ultimately in drinking water.

Bank filtration (BF) is a natural water treatment process which induces surface water to flow in response to a hydraulic gradient through sediment and into a vertical or horizontal well. It is a relatively cost-effective and robust technology. From a historical perspective, BF is first mentioned in the bible. In chapter 7 phrase 24 in Exodos, "all the Egyptians had to dig in the neighbourhood of the river for drinking water, since they could not drink the river water." BF has been recognized as a proven method for drinking water treatment in Europe. But these facilities have all been based on local experiences and thus far, there are no tools or a methodology that would help to transfer these experiences or the design and operation of a system from one place to another. Understanding the fate of effluent organic matter (EfOM) and natural organic matter (NOM) through BF is essential to assess the impact of wastewater effluent on the post treatment requirements of bank filtrates. Furthermore, their fate during drinking water treatment can significantly determine the process design.

Laboratory-scale batch and soil column experiments as well as analysis of the data from full-scale bank filtration and artificial recharge sites were conducted to obtain insight into the effect of source water quality (especially organic matter characteristics) and process conditions on the removal of organic micropollutants during soil passage. Wastewater effluent-impacted surface water and surface water were used as source waters in experiments with soil columns. Results showed the preferential removal of non-humic substances (i.e., biopolymers) from wastewater effluent-impacted surface water. The bulk organic matter characteristics of wastewater effluent-impacted surface water and surface water were similar after 5 m soil passage in laboratory column experiment. Humic-like organic matter in surface water and wastewater effluent-impacted surface water persisted through the soil passage. More than 50% of dissolved organic carbon (DOC) removal with significant reduction of dissolved oxygen (DO) was observed in the top 50 cm of the soil columns for both surface water and wastewater effluent-impacted surface water. This was due to biodegradation by soil biomass which was determined by adenosine triphosphate (ATP) concentrations and heterotrophic plate counts. Good correlation of DOC removal with DO and biomass development was observed in the soil columns.

Managed aquifer recharge (MAR) systems such as BF have been recognized as a multi-objective (-contaminant) barrier to provide safe drinking water by attenuating endocrine disrupting compounds (EDCs) and pharmaceutically active compounds (PhACs). In this thesis, the fate of selected EDCs and PhACs during soil passage was investigated. Firstly, estrogen compounds (i.e., EDCs) were tested to determine if these compounds can be attenuated during BF. Adsorption and biodegradation are the two important removal mechanisms for estrogen compounds (estrone, 17-estradiol and 17-ethinylestradiol), but adsorption exhibited to be the important removal mechanism. 17-estradiol and 17-ethinylestradiol were removed 99% and 96%, respectively, in batch experiment under oxic conditions. Biomass associated with sand and redox conditions did not show any significant effects on the removal of 17-estradiol. However, 17-ethinylestradiol removals varied from 64% to 87% in soil columns fed with different sources of water. Biodegradation appears to be more important in the removal of 17-ethinylestradiol. Estrogenic activity remaining under oxic conditions (13 ng estradiol-equivalents/L) was significantly lower than that of under anoxic conditions (97 ng estradiol-equivalents/L).

Secondly, batch studies were first conducted to investigate the removal of 13 selected PhACs from different water sources with respect to different sources of biodegradable organic matter. Column experiments were then performed to differentiate between biodegradation and sorption in the removal of these PhACs. Selected neutral PhACs (phenacetine, paracetamol and caffeine) and acidic PhACs (ibuprofen, fenoprofen, bezafibrate and naproxen) exhibited removal efficiencies of greater than 87% from different organic water matrices during batch studies (contact time: 60 days). In column studies, removal efficiencies of acidic PhACs (e.g., analgesics) decreased under biodegradable organic carbon-limited conditions. Removal efficiencies of selected acidic PhACs (ibuprofen, fenoprofen, bezafibrate, ketoprofen and naproxen) were less than 35% under abiotic conditions. These removals were attributed to sorption under abiotic conditions established by a biocide (20 mM of sodium azide), which suppressed microbial activity/biodegradation. However, under biotic conditions, removal efficiencies of these acidic PhACs compounds were greater than 78%, mainly attributed to biodegradation. Moreover, average removal efficiencies of hydrophilic (polar) neutral PhACs with low octanol/water partition coefficients (log K_{ow} < 2) (paracetamol, pentoxifylline, phenacetine and caffeine) were low (< 12 %) under abiotic conditions. However, under biotic conditions, removal efficiencies of selected neutral PhACs were greater than 91%. In contrast, carbamazepine showed a persistent behavior under both batch and column studies. Overall, results of this study showed that biodegradation is an important mechanism for removing PhACs during soil passage.

This study also analyzed a comprehensive database of OMPs at BF and artificial recharge (AR) field sites located near Lake Tegel in Berlin (Germany). The focus of the study was on the derivation of correlations between the removal efficiencies of OMPs and key factors influencing the performance of BF and AR. At the BF site, shallow monitoring wells located close to the Lake Tegel source exhibited oxic conditions followed by prolonged anoxic conditions in deep monitoring wells and a production well. At the AR site, oxic conditions prevailed from the recharge pond along monitoring wells up to the production well. Long residence times of up to 4.5 months at the BF site reduced the temperature variation during soil passage between summer and winter. The temperature variations were greater at the AR site as a consequence of shorter residence times. Deep monitoring wells and the production well located at the BF site were under the influence of ambient groundwater and old bank filtrate (up to several years of age). Thus, it is important to account for mixing with native groundwater and other sources (e.g., old bank filtrate) when estimating the performance of BF with respect to removal of OMPs. Principal component analysis (PCA) was used to investigate correlations between OMP removals and hydrogeochemical conditions with spatial and temporal parameters (e.g., well distance, residence time, and depth) from both sites. At the BF site, principal component-1 (PC1) embodied redox conditions (oxidation reduction potential and dissolved oxygen), and principal component-2 (PC2) embodied degradation potential (e.g., total organic carbon and dissolved organic carbon) and the calcium carbonate dissolution potential (Ca^{2+} and HCO_3^-). These two PCs explained a total variance of 55% at the BF site. At the AR site, PCA revealed redox conditions (PC1) and degradation potential with temperature (PC2) as principal components, which explained a total variance of 56%.

There is a need to develop assessment tools to help implement MAR as an effective barrier in attenuating different OMPs including PhACs and EDCs. In this study, guidelines were developed for different classes of OMPs, in which removal efficiencies of these compounds are determined as a function of travel times and distances. Guidelines are incorporated into Microsoft Excel spreadsheets and the water quality prediction tool was developed to estimate the removal of different classes of OMPs in MAR systems. Multiple linear regression analysis of data obtained from literature studies showed that travel (residence) time is one of the main parameters in estimating the performance of a MAR system for PhACs removal. Moreover, a quantitative structure activity relationship (QSAR) based model was proposed to predict OMP removals. The QSAR approach is especially useful for emerging compounds with little information about their fate during soil passage. Such an assessment framework for OMP removals is useful for adapting MAR as a multi-objective (-contaminant) barrier and understanding the fate of different classes of compounds during soil passage and the determination of post treatment requirements for MAR.

In general, this study showed that BF is an effective multiple objective barrier for removal of different contaminants present in surface water sources including organic micropollutants like PhACs and EDCs. The removal efficiencies of BF for these contaminants can be maximised by proper design of the recovery wells taking into consideration source water quality characteristics and local hydrogeological conditions.

Key words: artificial recharge, bank filtration, endocrine disrupting compounds, managed aquifer recharge, organic micropollutants, pharmaceutically active compounds, quantitative structure activity relationship.

Acknowledgements

First and foremost, I would like to express my sincere gratitude to my supervisor Prof. Gary Amy for it was his faith in my ability that offered an opportunity of Ph.D. study in UNESCO-IHE and TU-Delft. It was his guidance and encouragement which has made this thesis possible. I would also like to thank Dr. Sharma, who is my mentor, provided many helpful comments and supported me to finish my study. I would like to thank to Prof. J.C. van Dijk for advices and suggestions.

This study has been carried out within the framework of the European research project SWITCH (Sustainable Urban Water Management Improves Tomorrow's City's Health). SWITCH is supported by the European Commission under the 6th Framework Programme and contributes to the thematic priority area of "Global Change and Ecosystems" [1.1.6.3] Contract n° 018530-2. This study also partly supported by K-Water, UNESCO fellowship and Halla Energy and Environment. I would like to thank following MSc students for their supports (Mohammed Ibrahim, Emmanuel Ameda, Sharada Devkota, Henny Simarmata and Chol Abel). I want to express my great gratitude to Aleksandra Magic-Knezev, who helped me for allowing the use of advanced facilities in HetWaterlaboratorium. I would like to acknowledge the help of Theo van der Kaaij and Ineke van der Veer-Agterberg (HetWaterlaboratorium) for the support on LC-OCD/OND and ATP measurements. I want to express my gratitude to Dr. Gesche Grützmacher for advices and suggestions and the data from KWB Berlin. I want to thank Dr. Frank Sacher for analytical support for measuring pharmaceutically active compounds. I want to thank Karin Lekkerkerker for the support on translating samenvatting and proposition.

The members of UWS and laboratory staff in UNESCO-IHE have been a marvellous source of advices, supports, and ideas. Thanks go to Tanny van der Klis, Fred Kruis, Don van Galen, Peter Heerings, Lyzette Robbmont, Frank Widgman and Jolanda Boots. Special thanks should also go to the friends that maintained my sanity throughout Ph.D. study, Jongseop Choi, Denny Song, Sub Lee, Changwon Ha, Jungmin Lee, Patrick Yoo, Junghwan Kim, Gunjin Jung, Kyungsoo Kim, Victor Yangali, Sergio Rodríguez, Saeed Baghoth and Tarek Waly. I also thank to my colleagues from KIST, Dr. K-H Ahn, Dr. K.G. Song, Dr. S-H Lee, Dr. S-W Hong and Dr. G-P Kim. I want to express sincere gratitude the members of International Yi-Jun Memorial Church in the Netherlands and pastor C.K. Lee.

Last, but definitely not least, I would like to express my deepest thanks to my parents and brother, who helped me in every possible way. I could not end without expressing my gratitude to my daughters, Jusun and Juyeon, and my wife, Mikyoung. My two daughters born during my PhD study, and their supports allowed me to successfully finish my Ph.D. study. This thesis is dedicated to my father Sungyol Maeng who is in a hospital for cerebral infarction treatment.

Table of Contents

Chapter 1
INTRODUCTION

Summary

Many countries worldwide are faced with the challenge of providing safe drinking water to an ever-increasing population. Furthermore, increasing pollution of surface waters, often by wastewater effluent, has made water treatment much more difficult and expensive. Bank filtration (BF) is a managed aquifer recharge process which induces surface water to flow in response to a hydraulic gradient through sediment and into a vertical or horizontal recovery well. It is a relatively cost-effective and robust technology. From a historical perspective, BF is first mentioned in the bible. In chapter 7 phrase 24 in Exodos, "all the Egyptians had to dig in the neighborhood of the river for drinking water, since they could not drink the river water." BF has been recognized as a proven method for drinking water treatment in Europe. Removal of organic micropollutants, especially endocrine disrupting compounds, pharmaceutically active compounds, is a main concern in application of BF for water treatment. The mechanism of their removal during soil passage and the associated influential factors are not fully understood. Therefore, this study aims to analyze the effect of source water quality and the process conditions applied on the removal of organic micropollutants during BF.

1.1. Bank filtration

As the world population is increasing, provision of clean drinking water is become an important global environmental problem around the world, especially in developing countries. Many water utilities in developed countries have been employing advanced water treatment methods like membrane filtration or advanced oxidation. But in developing countries, most water utilities have conventional treatment processes or less, and there is lack of financial resources and manpower for advanced treatment technologies. Many developing countries discharge their sewage into the receiving aquatic environment without any treatment or after only primary treatment. Therefore, the contaminant loadings are higher than that of developed countries so advanced methods (e.g., membrane filtration and advanced oxidation) may not remove all the contaminants as designed.

Bank filtration (BF) has been recognized as a proven method for drinking water treatment process in Europe. The inhabitants of Düsseldorf (approximately 600,000 people) have been supplied with drinking water through BF in the Rhine River for 130 years (Eckert and Irmscher, 2006). Also, more than 100 BF sites in Europe have been using BF as a drinking water treatment process and several wells have been operated for more than 100 years (Irmscher and Teermann, 2002). In the United States, BF is considered as a pre-treatment process for removing microbial pathogens but does not receive as much credit by regulators as in European countries. However, the use of BF systems by water utilities has increased because of their effectiveness and sustainability around the world.

Aquifer passage and infiltration are considered essential components of BF and artificial recharge (AR). AR is commonly applied in reclamation of wastewater effluent reuse (i.e., soil aquifer treatment, (SAT)). This technique involves the infiltration of water into the aquifer through infiltration basin or direct injection through one or more injection wells. Later, the same wells or pumping wells are used for recovery of filtrate water. The performance of these systems is mainly dictated by redox conditions, and the hydraulic conductivity of an aquifer plays a key role in determining yield. In a BF system, riverbank filtration (RBF) and lake bank filtration (LBF) are commonly used, and there are some differences between RBF, LBF and AR (Table 1.1): the selective intake and pretreatment (AR), rehabilitation of riverbed hydraulic conductivity (AR), travelling distance and residence time (RBF, LBF>AR), and oxic condition (AR> RBF, LBF).

Table 1.1 Characteristics of RBF, LBF and AR sites

Parameter	RBF/LBF sites	AR site
Residence time	Longer (>3 months)	Shorter (>50 days)
Selective intake and pretreatment	No	Yes
Redox conditions	Short oxic zone followed by a more reduced zone	Mainly oxic zone
Temperature change (season)	Lower (12 – 15°C)	Higher (20 - 25°C)
Temperature influence	Less influence of temperature on redox conditions	Higher influence of temperature leading to seasonal changes in redox conditions

Sources: Maeng et al. (2010); Grünheid et al. (2005)

BF is a sustainable technology for water treatment if the system is designed and operated with proper guidelines in an appropriate hydrogeological location because the sediment layer of the subsurface, redox conditions and the travel time play an important role in the performance of BF system (Figure 1.1). Thus, a feasibility assessment including preliminary pumping tests is often necessary to determine the most suitable location of the production well. However, a pumping test is time consuming and requires some costs. Currently, several groundwater modeling software packages are available to predict the yield of BF at user selected locations. However, a decision tool which is able to predict the optimum location of a well with respective of water quality is not available.

4

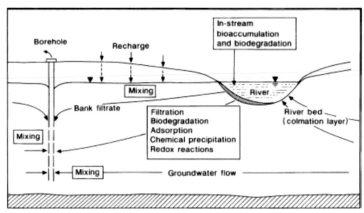

Sources: Hiscock and Grischek (2002)

Figure 1.1 Schematic diagram of a bank filtration system

A managed aquifer recharge (MAR) system such as BF is attractive for drinking water production not only for developing countries but also for developed countries because it can cope with extreme variations in water quality and can efficiently deal with chemical shock loads or temperature changes. In many cases a BF can serve as a pre-treatment which is following by advanced treatment processes to improve the water quality further, thus reducing the overall cost of water treatment. However, only a few studies have been done on infiltration of polluted surface water (Ćosović et al., 1996; Reemtsma et al., 2000). The effects from effluent organic matter on the fate organic micropollutants derived from wastewater effluent during BF are not fully understood.

1.2. Pharmaceutically active compounds and endocrine disrupting compounds in the receiving aquatic environment

1.2.1. Pharmaceutically active compounds

Recently, the occurrence and fate of pharmaceutically active compounds (PhACs) in the receiving aquatic environment has gained much interest from scientists and public. The U.S. Geological Survey conducted a nationwide occurrence study on streams and rivers under the influence of secondary effluent and agricultural runoff, and the study showed that a large number of trace organic pollutants which can have an adverse impact on public health can be present in surface water and ground water (Kolpin et al., 2002). A study done by Heberer (2002b) revealed that more than 80 PhACs and several drug metabolites were detected in the aquatic environment of following countries: Austria, Brazil, Canada, Croatia, England, Germany, Greece, Italy, Spain and Switzerland. Most of the PhACs are not completely taken up by the human body and some (i.e., metabolites) are excreted into municipal wastewater in their original form or in a slightly metabolized form (Heberer, 2002a).

Analgesics and anti-inflammatory compounds are often detected in secondary effluent. The study done by Heberer (2002b) showed that PhACs such as clofibric acid, diclofenac, ibuprofen, propyphenazone, primidone, gemfibrozil, naproxen, ketoprofen and carbamazepine were detected at individual concentrations up to the μg/L-level in the effluents from sewage treatment plants (STPs) in Berlin, Germany. PhACs in secondary effluent could reach the surface waters and subsequently to ground water by soil aquifer treatment or naturally occurring infiltration into an aquifer. According to the previous study, the drinking water treatment plant located downstream of a sewage treatment plant provided water that contained 8 ng/L of ibuprofen and ketoprofen during winter time (Vieno et al., 2005). Even though PhACs and their metabolites are present in aquatic environments, scientists believe that at the low levels of PhACs in the aquatic environment do not pose an appreciable risk to human health (Schwab, 2005). However, the possible detrimental effects of PhACs on the aquatic environment and lifelong exposure are currently not well known and especially for those PhACs recently developed (Cunningham et al., 2006).

1.2.2. Endocrine disrupting compounds

The use of organic chemicals has been increasing over the last four decades and consequently it has led to abnormalities in the aquatic environment (Blaber, 1970; Gomes and Lester, 2003; Smith, 1971). Endocrine disrupting compounds (EDCs) in aquatic environments interfere with endocrine glands and their hormones or where the hormones act – the target tissues. Many EDCs have non-polar and hydrophobic characteristics and are favorably absorbed onto particulates. Therefore, most of EDCs are often concentrated in suspended solids or sediment rather than in the aqueous phase, and the intrusion of EDCs into ground water is minimized by subsurface characteristics so ground water is less influenced by EDCs to travel compared to surface waters. However, sediments can be dynamic under seasonal variations, enabling bound EDCs for long distances into an aquifer. Therefore, the degradation kinetics of bound EDCs is important to investigate and it is dependent on numerous factors: redox conditions, temperature, dissolved organic matter and pH. Figure 1.2 shows sources and behavior of EDCs in the receiving aquatic environment.

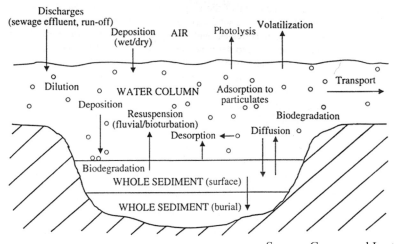

Source: Gomes and Lester (2003)

Figure 1.2 Sources and behaviour of EDCs in the receiving aquatic environment.

Among many EDCs, estrogens such as estrone (E1), 17β-estradiol (E2) and 17α-ethinylestradiol (EE2) showed the most estrogenic activity, and alkylphenols (APs) and their ethoxylates (APEOs) showed less than that of estrogens (Gomes and Lester, 2003). With advances in technology and instrumentation, estrogens can now be measured more accurately in the range of parts per trillion (ppt) and there is an increasing concern about the presence of those EDCs in the aquatic environment (Shappell, 2006). Ternes et al (1999) showed the frequent presence of E1 and E2 in effluent of German and Canadian STPs over ranges of ng/L, with a maximum concentration of 70 ng/L for E1. Recently, several studies showed the presence of estrogens in surface waters, wastewater and treated wastewater in different parts of the world (Carballa et al., 2004; Cargouët et al., 2004; Hintemann et al., 2006; Lishman et al., 2006; Ma et al., 2007; Nakada et al., 2005; Sarmah et al., 2006). A number of studies have reported that the feminization of male aquatic species in receiving waters mainly originated from the effluents from wastewater treatment plants, and surface runoff from agricultural activities and municipal biosolids (Khanal et al., 2006). It is plausible that EDCs exposure could be harmful to humans and may be a reason for some of the increases in human disorders. There is a need to understand the biodegradability, sorption and transport of estrogen compounds (E1, E2 and EE2) during BF. Therefore, understanding the fate of those estrogens during BF provides insight into development of a model which help to predict estrogen removals during soil passage.

1.3. Problem identification

Most BF systems located in Europe and the USA have been successfully implemented as natural filtration systems to produce high drinking water quality. For example, in Berlin, after abstraction, aeration and rapid sand filtration are the only treatment before distribution (no final disinfection). The environmental conditions in which BF systems operate in North America and European countries are favorable such as high quality source water with many experiences in designing BF systems. However, it is not always true for many industrialized Asian countries and developing countries where a river often carries tremendous amounts of a sewage load. Moreover, hydrogeological information is unknown, and ground water is often polluted. Several studies were carried out to determine the performance of soil passage on polluted surface water in both field and laboratory studies (Ćosović et al., 1996; Jekel and Gruenheid, 2005; Reemtsma et al., 2000). However, the potential implications of running a BF system under extreme environmental conditions (i.e., wastewater effluent-impacted surface water) with respect to the fate of bulk organic matter, EDCs and PhACs is not well known.

Many studies have shown that BF is a promising technology for pre-treatment of raw water prior to conventional water treatment by removing bulk organic matter and trace organic contaminants including PhACs and EDCs and reducing the cost of chemicals (Grünheid et al., 2005; Heberer et al., 2003; Maeng et al., 2008; Schmidt et al 2007). However, the performance of BF in removing those contaminants depends on several factors including hydraulic conductivity, temperature, redox conditions and travel time, and there is a lack of fundamental understanding of the mechanism of degradation of bulk organic matter and organic micropollutants under different redox conditions during BF.

So far, there are no design guidelines, tools/software or simulators that help to transfer the experiences or design of BF system from one place to another. BF has been successfully applied for water treatment in Europe and the United States, and many water utilities companies have a great interest in BF as a new source of water supply. However, existing BF facilities have all been based on local experiences. For water supply companies, currently there are no tools or guidelines for the design of BF systems and to predict the fate of PhACs or EDCs during soil passage. Therefore, a modeling framework and guidelines are necessary to serve as a screening tool to estimate the water quality from a BF system before conducting costly pilot experiments and site investigations. Therefore, this research is an innovative effort to better understand and utilize the multi-objectives water treatment potential of BF.

1.4. Research hypothesis and objectives

1.4.1. Hypothesis

Four hypotheses have been developed based on a literature survey. Each hypothesis is elaborated below along with a brief statement supporting its development.

(i) Biodegradable components of effluent organic matter (EfOM) found in wastewater effluent can be effectively removed during BF and will promote degradation of EDCs and PhACs. The role of EfOM in BF can be verified using laboratory-scale soil column studies. Both EfOM and NOM show heterogeneity with respect to organic fractions and they can be characterized by molecular weight distribution, size exclusion chromatography, specific ultraviolet absorbance, fluorescence and carbon-13 nuclear magnetic resonance spectroscopy (Drewes et al., 2006). EfOM has a greater biodegradable organic carbon fraction than that of naturally derived organic matter according to preliminary experiments (results not shown). Therefore, more viable biomass and diversity of microorganism distributions attached to soil can enhance the degradation of bulk organic matter. Biodegradable dissolved organic carbon (BDOC) limits soil biomass growth during soil infiltration of conventionally treated effluents (Rauch-Williams and Drewes, 2006). The removal of different organic fractions (NOM, EfOM, glucose and glutamic acid) has shown a positive correlation with respect to total viable biomass in column studies (Rauch and Drewes, 2005).

(ii) The variation in bulk organic matter and redox conditions affect biomass activity in removing estrogenic compounds during BF. The degradation of free estrogen compounds mainly involves biodegradation but, in biotic column studies, estrogen concentrations high enough to cause the detrimental effect on endocrine systems in aquatic environments still remained under abiotic conditions (DEPA, 2004). The biodegradation fraction of bulk organic matter will be a limiting factor in the biomass development, and total viable biomass will play an important role in degrading estrogen compounds. More estrogen compounds are degraded at higher concentrations of biosolids (Ternes et al., 1999). Therefore, total viable biomass in soil may vary the degradation rate of estrogens. Also, changes in redox conditions during BF may significantly influence the degradation kinetics of organic micropollutants including estrogens. In many cases E2 could be readily transformed to E1, however, the complete degradation of estrogen compounds under anoxic conditions was minimal (Czajka and Londry, 2006). During BF, if dissolved oxygen is rapidly depleted, estrogens may accumulate in the aquifer because of their potential to be recalcitrant under anoxic conditions. The redox conditions may drive the fate of estrogen compounds in the environment and impact both the rates and mechanisms of estrogen compound transformation.

(iii) The removal of PhACs during BF can be optimized by controlling redox conditions. A recent study showed the effect of variable redox conditions on the behavior of a number of PhACs including carbamazepine, phenazone, and several phenazone-type PhACs (Massmann et al., 2006). In this study, oxygen concentration changes in infiltrate throughout the season affected the removal of PhACs, and the role of oxygen presence during BF was more decisive than the temperature dependency. During winter, when oxygen concentrations were high in infiltrate, the removal of phenazone-type pharmaceuticals was more efficient than summer. Phenazone-type pharmaceuticals are as redox sensitive PhACs and are able to be fully degraded during winter when oxygen concentration is high. Temperature is known as an influential growth parameter for bacteria, and water temperatures during summer may increase the growth activity of phenazone-degrading bacteria during winter. However, redox conditions play a more important role for phenazone-degrading bacteria in removing phenazone-type pharmaceuticals. Conversely, Vieno et al. (2005) showed that cold seasons (low temperature) can severely increase the environmental risk of pharmaceuticals (ibuprofen, naproxen, ketoprofen, diclofenac, and bezafibrate) and the risk for contamination of drinking water because the elimination of the PhACs decreased significantly in a sewage treatment plant (STP) (an average of 25% compared to spring and summer) in wintertime, leading to increased concentrations of PhACs in the effluent water. A drinking water treatment plant (DWTP) located downstream from a STP has a high risk of PhACs in their produced water. In this case, employing a BF system may prevent the introduction of PhACs into the DWTP. Further investigation is required for other PhACs in order to conclude that the role of oxygen presence is more decisive than temperature in removing PhACs during BF. Experiments on biodegradability of emerging PhACs under different redox conditions should be used to advance the prediction tools for BF systems and enable management of the risk of PhACs in BF infiltrate. However, there have been very limited studies done in the prediction of PhACs from BF.

(iv) A modeling framework provides a means of assessing the operational variables in order to obtain an optimal configuration of BF systems with respect to required bulk organic matter, EDCs and PhACs removal efficiencies. The reported removals of dissolved organic carbon, nitrogen-species and selected organic micropollutants during BF will be analyzed using statistical techniques such as multiple regression and principal component analysis, and simple first or zero order expressions applied to develop time-distance relationships in order to delineate removal trends as a function of site characteristics and operating conditions.

1.4.2. Objectives

Based on the literature survey above, the following are the specific objectives of this study.

1) To evaluate changes in the fate of bulk organic matter based on soil column studies which simulate the impact of wastewater effluent during BF

2) To investigate the fate of EDCs (estrogen compounds) during BF

3) To investigate the fate of selected PhACs during BF

4) To analyze removals of selected organic micropollutants with hydrogeochemical conditions and spatial parameters using principal component analysis (PCA) in order to statistically delineate removal trends at BF and AR sites.

5) To develop a modeling framework for the assessment and prediction of treated water quality from a BF system, especially focusing on organic micropollutants

1.5. References

Birkett., J.W., 2003. Sources of endocrine disrupter: London, IWS Publishing & Lewis Publishers.

Blaber, S.J.M., 1970. The occurrence of a penis-like outgrowth behind the right tentacle in spent females of Nucella lapillus: Proc. Malac. Soc. London, 39, 231-233.

Carballa, M., Omil, F., Lema, J.M., Llompart, M., García-Jares, C., Rodríguez, I., Gómez, M. and Ternes, T., 2004. Behavior of pharmaceuticals, cosmetics and hormones in a sewage treatment plant, Water Res. 38, 2918-2926.

Cargouët, M., Peridiz, D., Mouatassim-Souali, A., Tamisier-Karolak, S. and Levi, Y., 2004. Assessment of river contamination by estrogenic compounds in Paris area (France), Sci. Total Environ. 324, 55-66.

Colborn, T. and Clement, C., 1992 Chemically induced alteration in sexual development: the wildlife/human connection.: Princeton NJ, Princeton Scientific Publishing Company.

Ćosović, B., Hršak, D., Vojvodić, V. and Krznarić, D., 1996. Transformation of organic matter and bank filtration from a polluted stream, Water Res. 30, 2921-2928.

Cunningham, V.L., Bunzy, M., Hutchinson, T., Mastrocco, F., Parke, N. and Roden, N., 2006. Effects of human pharmacetuicals on aquatic life: next step, Environ. Sci. Technol. 40, 3456-3462.

Czajka, C.P. and Londry, K.L., 2006. Anaerobic biotransformation of estrogens, Sci. Total Environ. 367, 932-941.

DEPA, 2004. Degradation of estrogens in sewage treatment processes. Danish Environmental Protection Agency.

Drewes, J.E., Quanrud, D.M., Amy, G.L. and Westerhoff, P.K., 2006. Character of organic matter in soil-aquifer treatment system. J. Environ. Eng. 132(11), 1447-1458.

Eckert, P. and Irmscher, R., 2006. Practical Paper Over 130 years of experience with Riverbank Filtration in Dussldorf, Germany, J. Water Supply Res. T. AQUA. 55, 283-291.

Gomes, R.L. and Lester, J.N., 2003. Endocrine Disrupters in Receiving Waters, London, IWA Publishing & Lewis Publishers.

Grünheid, S., Amy, G., and Jekel, M., 2005. Removal of bulk dissolved organic carbon (DOC) and trace organic compounds by bank filtration and artificial recharge. Water Res. 39 (14), 3219.

Hanselman, T.A., Graetz, D.A., and Wilkie, A.C., 2003. Manure-Borne estrogens as potential environmental contaiminants: A review, Environ. Sci. Technol. 37, 5471-5478.

Heberer, T., 2002a. Occurrence, fate, and removal of pharmaceutical residues in the aquatic environment: a review of recent research data, Toxicol. Lett., 131, 5-17.

Heberer, T., 2002b. Tracking persistent pharmaceutical residues from municipal sewage to drinking water, J. Hydrol., 266, 175-189.

Heberer, T., Mechlinski, A., and Fanck, B., 2003. NASRI - Occurrence and Fate of Pharmaceuticals during Bank Filtration In Conference Wasser Berlin 2003, Berlin, Germany.

Hintemann, T., Schneider, C., Schöler, H. and Schneider, R., 2006. Field study using two immunoasays for the determination of estadiol and ethinylestradiol in the aquatic environment, Water Res. 40, 2287-2294.

Hiscock, K. M. amd Grischek, T. 2002. Attenuation of groundwater pollution by bank filtration. J. Hydrol., 266 (3-4) 139-144.

Irmscher, R. and Teermann, I., 2002. Riverbank filtration for drinking water supply - a proven method, perfect to face today's challenge, Water Sci. Technol., 2, 1-8.

Jekel, M. and Gruenheid, S., 2005. Bank filtration and grounwater recharge for treatment of polluted surface waters, Wat. Sci. Tech., 5, 57-66.

Khanal, S.K., Xie, B., Thompson, M.L., Sung, S., Ong, S.-K. and Leeuwen, J.V., 2006. Fate, and transport and biodegradation of natural estrogens in the environment and engineerin systems, Environ. Sci. Technol., 40, 6537-6545.

Kolpin, D.W., Furlong, E.T., Meyer, M.T., Thurman, E.M., Zaugg, S.D., Barber, L.B. and Buxton, H.T., 2002. Pharmaceuticals, Hormones, and Other Organic Wastewater Contaminants in U.S. Streams, 1999-2000: A National Reconnaissance, Environ. Sci. Technol. 36, 1202-1211.

Lishman, L., Smyth, S.A., Sarafin, K., Kleywegt, S., Toito, J., Peart, T., Lee, B., Servos, M., Beland, M., and Seto, P., 2006. Occurrence and reductions of pharmaceuticals and personal care products and estrogens by municipal wastewater treatment plants in Ontario, Canada, Sci. Total Environ., 367.

Ma, M., Rao, K. and Wang, Z., 2007. Occurrence of estrogenic effects in sewage and industrial wastewaters in Beijing, China. Environmental Pollution 147(2), 331-336.

Maeng, S. K., Sharma, S. K., Amy, G. and Magic-Knezev, A., 2008. Fate of effluent organic matter (EfOM) and natural organic matter (NOM) through riverbank filtration. Water Sci. Technol. 57(12), 1999–2007.

S.K. Maeng, S.K., Ameda, E.A., Sharma, S.K. , Grützmacher, G. and Amy, G.L. 2010. Organic micropollutant removal from wastewater effluent-impacted drinking water sources during bank filtration and artificial recharge. Water Res. 44 (11), 4003-4014.

Massmann, G., Greskowiak, J., Dünnbier, U. and Zuehlke, S., 2006. The impact of variable temeratures on the redox conditions and the behavior of pharmaceutical residues during artifical recharge. J. Hydrol. 328(1-2), 141-156.

Nakada, N., Yasojima, M., Miyajima, K., Komori, K., Suzuki, Y. and Tanaka, H., 2005. Fate of estrogenic compounds and estrogenic activity in wastewater treatment process, Technology 2nd Joint Specialty Conference for Sustainable Management of Water Quality Systems for the 21st Century: Working to Project Public Health, Water Environment Federation: San Francisco, USA, 298-304.

Rauch, T. and Drewes, J.E., 2006. Using soil biomass as an indicator for the biological removal of effluent-derived organic carbon during soil infiltration. Water Res., 40,961-068.

Reemtsma, T., Gnirß, R. and Jekel, M., 2000. Infiltration of combined sewer overflow and tertiary municipal wastewater: An intergrated laboratory and field study on nutrients and dissolved organics, Water. Res., 34, 1179-1186.

Sarmah, A.K., Northcott, G.L., Leusch, F.D.L. and Tremblay, L.A., 2006. A study of endocrine disrupting chemicals (EDCs) in municipal sewage and amimal waste effluents in the Waikato region of New Zealand, Sci. Total Environ., 355, 135-144.

Schmidt, C. K., Lange, F. T. and Brauch, H. J., 2007.Characteristics and evaluation of natural attenuation processes for organic micropollutant removal during riverbank filtration. In Regional IWA conference on groundwater management in the Danube River Basin and other large River Basins, 7-9 June 2007, 231-236 Belgrade, Serbia.

Shappell, N.W., 2006. Estrogenic activity in the environment: muniicipal wastewater effluent, river, ponds and wetlands, J. Environ. Qual.35, 122-132.

Smith, B.S., 1971. Sexuality in the American mud snail, Nassarius obsoletus, Proc. Malac. Soc. London, 39, 377-378.

Ternes, T.A., Stumpf, M., Mueller, J., Haberer, K. and Wilken, R.-D., 1999. Behavior and occurrence of estrogens in municipal sewage treatment plant - I. Investigations in Germany, Canada and Brazil. Sci. Total Environ., 225, 81-90.

Vieno, N.M., Tuhkanen, T. and Kronberg, L., 2005. Seasonal Variation in the Occurrence of Pharmaceuticals in Effluents from a Sewage Treatment Plant and in the Recipient Water, Environ. Sci. Technol. 39, 8220-8226.

Chapter 2

OCCURRENCE AND FATE OF BULK ORGANIC MATTER AND PHARMACEUTICALLY ACTIVE COMPOUNDS IN MANAGED AQUIFER RECHARGE

Parts of this chapter were based on:

Maeng, S.K., Sharma, S.K, Lekkerkerker, K., Amy, G.L., Occurrence and fate of bulk organic matter and pharmaceutically active compounds in managed aquifer recharge, Submitted to Water Research.

14

Summary

Detailed characteristics of bulk organic matter and the occurrence and fate of pharmaceutically active compounds (PhACs) during through managed aquifer recharge (MAR) such as bank filtration (BF) and artificial recharge (AR) were reviewed. Understanding the fate of bulk organic matter through BF and AR is essential to determine the pre- and/or post-treatment requirements. Analysis of organic matter characteristic using a suite of analytical tools suggests that there is a preferential removal of non-humic substances during MAR. Different classes of PhACs were found to behave differently during BF and AR. Antibiotics, non-steroidal anti-inflammatory drugs (NSAIDs), beta blockers and steroid hormones generally exhibited good removal efficiencies. However, anticonvulsants showed a persistent behavior during soil passage. There were also some redox dependent PhACs. For example, X-Ray contrast agents, determined as adsorbable organic iodine (AOI), and sulfamethoxazole (antibiotics) degraded more favorably under anoxic conditions compared to oxic conditions. Phenazone-type pharmaceuticals (NSAIDs) exhibited a better removal under oxic conditions. The redox transition from oxic to anoxic conditions during soil passage can enhance the removal of PhACs that are sensitive to redox conditions. In general, BF and AR can potentially be included in a multi-barrier treatment system for the removal of PhACs.

2.1. Introduction

Bulk organic matter in natural waters mainly consists of naturally organic matter (NOM), derived from allochthonous and autochthonous sources. NOM does not pose a direct health threat to humans with respect to drinking water quality, but it is a precursor of organic disinfection by-products (DBP). In wastewater effluent-impacted (or effluent-dominated) surface waters, bulk organic matter is a mixture of NOM and effluent organic matter (EfOM) which originates from wastewater treatment plants. While EfOM has not been extensively studied compared to NOM, EfOM is composed of different types of organics: refractory compounds, residual degradable substrate, intermediates, complex organic compounds, and soluble microbial products (SMPs) (Barker and Stuckey, 1999). SMPs are biodegradable organic matter produced from substrate metabolism and biomass decay, and are known as major foulants for reverse osmosis (RO), nano filtration (NF), and ultra filtration (UF) membranes (Jarusutthirak and Amy, 2006). Moreover, SMPs are precursor materials of nitrogenous disinfection by-products (N-DBPs) and can lead to bacterial regrowth in drinking water distribution systems (Amy and Drewes, 2007).

EfOM also consists of emerging contaminants such as pharmaceutically active compounds (PhACs), endocrine disrupting compounds (EDCs), and personal care products (PCPs). The main route of PhACs and transformation products into surface water is through discharged effluent from wastewater treatment plants as result of patient excretion by both urine and feces (Cunningham et al., 2006; Zhou et al., 2009). Previous studies done by Kasprzyk-Hordern et al. (2009) and Zhou et al. (2009) showed the impact of wastewater effluent containing organic micropollutants (OMPs) (e.g., PhACs) on the quality of receiving waters. Non-point sources such as overland flow (i.e., runoff) during rainfall or land drainage in agriculture areas also deliver PhACs (e.g., veterinary medicines) to surface water or groundwater (Boxall et al., 2004). This therefore creates the possibility for the occurrence of OMPs such as PhACs, PCPs, and EDCs in drinking water sources.

Currently, the total consumption of PhACs and PCPs in the world is not known because many of these compounds significantly vary with respect to application and consumption from one country to another (Cunningham, 2004). Many of them are slightly transformed or unchanged during municipal wastewater treatment (Chefetz et al., 2008). Moreover, the growing use of PhACs, EDCs, and PCPs for human and veterinary purposes has contributed to their frequent detection in the aquatic environment and wastewater (Heberer, 2002; Tixier et al., 2003; Jjemba, 2006). Growing concern over the safety of drinking water from PhACs, EDCs and PCPs has resulted in increased research worldwide (Mechlinski and Heberer, 2005; Kim et al., 2007; Kümmerer, 2009; Madden et al., 2009; Mompelat et al., 2009). Many water utilities in developed countries are adapting advanced water treatment processes to provide a reliable supply of safe drinking water. However, little is known about the fate of transformation products formed in drinking water treatment processes (e.g., advanced oxidation processes (AOPs) and biodegradation) (Mompelat et al., 2009).

Snyder et al. (2007) evaluated the removal of EDCs and PhACs in 13 full-scale water treatment facilities. Conventional coagulation, flocculation and sedimentation processes were inefficient for removing most of target EDCs and PCPs. Slow sand filtration and flocculation by iron (III) chloride were also inefficient for selected pharmaceuticals (bezafibrate, clofibric acid, carbamazepine and diclofenac) (Ternes et al., 2002). However, AOPs (e.g., UV/H_2O_2 and ozone/H_2O_2) were highly effective for removing many OMPs (Gebhardt and Schröer, 2007; Snyder et al., 2007; Klavarioti et al., 2009). NF and RO membrane systems have been known as effective processes for removing pharmaceutical residues (Yoon et al., 2006; Yangali-Quintanilla et al., 2009). Radjenovic et al. (2008) demonstrated that NF and RO membranes appeared to be very efficient in most of pharmaceutical residues in a full-scale drinking water treatment plant. However, construction and maintenance costs for both membrane and AOPs systems are limiting factors in the implementation of a large treatment facility. Retrofitting conventional water treatment facilities with membrane or AOP systems to remove pharmaceutical residues is also relatively costly, thus leading to a high unit treatment cost of water which makes water unaffordable. In contrast to a high-cost system, managed aquifer recharge (MAR) processes (e.g., bank filtration (BF) and artificial recharge (AR)) are robust and cost-effective systems for organic micropollutant (OMP) removal.

BF and AR systems are often adapted by water utilities where their raw water quality (e.g., surface water) is not good enough or the amount of raw water (e.g., groundwater) is not sufficient. Often, water utilities with BF and AR are located downstream from municipal wastewater treatment plants, especially for those water utilities which use a river that flows through many cities or countries (e.g., Rhine River, Germany). In this case, it is nearly impossible to withdraw raw water without any impact of wastewater effluent, and the fraction of wastewater effluent in the river can be varied. For example, BF facilities located in Berlin, Germany are managed by Berlin Water Works (Berliner Wasserbetriebe), and their source water (Lake Tegel) is influenced by well-treated domestic wastewater effluent between 15 and 30% (Jekel and Grünheid, 2005; Pekdeger, 2006). Ćosović et al. (1996) investigated a BF site (Zagreb, Croatia) under extreme conditions where chemical oxygen demand (COD) of surface water was several thousand mg O_2/L, most of which is biodegradable organic matter from a local yeast industry and from the pharmaceutical industry for the production of antibiotics and synthetic organic compounds. If source water for BF and AR systems contains EfOM that originates from a wastewater treatment plant, it is necessary to assess the characteristics of bulk organic matter and the fate of pharmaceuticals and transformation products for the pre- and/or post-treatment requirements of BF and AR.

In this Chapter, the occurrence and removal of bulk organic matter and PhACs are evaluated for MAR systems (i.e., BF and AR). Moreover, the fate of bulk organic matter and PhACs for BF and AR systems is also addressed. This study collected and reviewed data from full-scale studies carried out at BF and AR field sites around the world, and data from laboratory-scale and pilot studies were used if no data were available from BF and AR field sites.

2.2. Managed aquifer recharge systems: bank filtration and artificial recharge

BF is a robust and cost effective treatment technology that has been proven to be an excellent option for the attenuation of OMPs often found in surface waters (Schmidt et al. 2007). This technology has several advantages over (direct) surface water intake because of its capability to remove suspended solids, biodegradable organic matter, bacteria, viruses, parasites, partial elimination of adsorbable compounds through mixing, biodegradation and sorption (Hiscock and Grischek, 2002). Water utilities in the Netherlands and some in Germany, using BF or AR as a water treatment process, have been supplying drinking water without a disinfection process (chlorine). This does not apply to all BF sites because of source water qualities (river/lake), hydrogeological conditions, residence times and travel distances are different between sites (i.e., site specific). Recently, BF and AR have become an attractive process as part of a protective multi-barrier treatment of emerging contaminants (e.g., PhACs, PCPs, and EDCs) and also reduce organic/biological fouling of membrane systems (Nederlof et al., 2000; Speth et al., 2002). BF has been shown to be a robust system against chemical spills or accidents by damping the pollutants through sorption, biodegradation and mixing (Ray et al., 2002c; Schmidt et al., 2007). All of these benefits make MAR systems like BF and AR more attractive.

The hydraulic gradient between the river/lake/infiltration basin and a production well is created by pumping from the production well, and the gradient induces infiltrated water from river/lake/infiltration basin towards a production well(s) resulting in a mixture of groundwater originally in the aquifer and the infiltrated water from the river/lake/infiltration basin (Schmidt et al., 2003). Naturally, during flooding conditions, the elevated level of river water move towards the aquifer under non-pumping conditions (Ray et al., 2002c). The degree of hydraulic connection between surface waters and the aquifer is an important factor that decides the feasibility of the process and location of a pumping well(s).

MAR processes have been studied and practiced in (1) Europe (Bourg and Bertin, 1993; Hiscock and Grischek, 2002; Irmscher and Teermann, 2002; Hiemstra et al., 2003; Eckert and Irmscher, 2006; Kedziorek et al., 2008); (2) North America (Ray et al., 2002b; Gupta et al., 2009); (3) Africa (Shamrukh and Abdel-Wahab, 2008); and (4) Asia (Lee et al., 2009; Wu et al., 2007). BF has been applied for over a century in some parts of Central Europe, especially Germany (Irmscher and Teermann, 2002; Ray et al., 2002a; Tufenkji et al., 2002; Jekel and Grünheid, 2003; Eckert and Irmscher, 2006; Ray, 2008). It is a popular treatment process in Europe (Germany, Netherlands, France and Hungary), with 70% of MAR sites (BF and AR) located in Europe followed by North America (23%), Asia (4%), Australia (2%) and Africa (1%) (Grützmacher et al., 2009). In Europe, BF and AR are considered as a major part of drinking water treatment; but in North America, BF and AR have been applied mainly as a pre-treatment step to save on treatment costs due to lower chemical and energy requirements for removal of contaminants like pathogens, particles, suspended matter and some dissolved organic carbon (Grünheid et al., 2005). BF or AR sites in North America and Europe have generally favorable conditions such as high quality of source water (e.g., river and lake) and location at a site with well-defined hydrogeological conditions. However, this is not always true for many developing countries where a river is often contaminated by wastes from many different sources (e.g., agricultural runoff and municipal wastewaters) and lack of hydrogeological information.

2.3. Physicochemical properties of pharmaceutically active compounds

As surface water infiltrates through the riverbed sediments and aquifer materials, most suspended solids, biodegradable organic compounds and other contaminants are removed (Ray, 2008). The main attenuation mechanisms of PhACs for MAR processes are biodegradation and sorption. Biodegradation and sorption are considered to be important mechanisms during soil passage (Schoenheinz et al., 2005). However, some polar and refractory PhACs are often detected in infiltrated water, necessitating monitoring of their fate and mobility, and their levels are often highly dependent on the physicochemical properties of PhACs. For proper understanding of PhACs removal during soil passage, the role of physicochemical properties of PhACs with respect to biodegradation and sorption must be well understood.

2.3.1. Effect of PhACs properties on biodegradation in managed aquifer recharge

The complete conversion of organic compounds into inorganic products (i.e., mineralization) in waters and soils is mostly due to microbial activity (Alexander, 1981). Therefore, the potential of PhACs to be biotransformed or mineralized (i.e., ultimate biodegradation) is an important aspect of their fate during soil passage. Both chemical structures and physicochemical properties significantly impact the degree of biodegradation during soil passage. The relative biodegradability of an organic compound based on structural properties was summarized by Howard (2000). This study summarized 7 different structural properties (e.g., branching, aliphatic functional groups, aromatic functional groups, aliphatic amines, halophenols, polycyclic aromatics, and triazines) that determine the biodegradability of a compound. For example, electron withdrawing aromatic substituents such as nitro groups and halogens aromatic substituents decrease biodegradability and make it more difficult for enzymes to degrade a compound. In contrast, the aromatic substituents with donating functionalities (e.g., carboxylic acids and amines) increase biodegradability (Howard, 2000).

2.3.2. Effect of PhACs properties on sorption in managed aquifer recharge

The removal of PhACs by sorption is also an important mechanism during soil passage, contributing to compound attenuation. The organic carbon partition coefficient, K_{oc}, is often used to assess the sorption and distribution behavior of non-polar OMPs in soils/sediments. The organic carbon content of soil/sediment greatly contributes to the sorption of non-polar PhACs (e.g., pesticides and industrial chemicals). However, K_{oc} may not properly describe the distribution behavior between soil and water for some PhACs which contain charged sites and exist as an ionic compound in the aquatic environment (Cunningham, 2004). Ionic interactions become a key factor in sorption mechanisms for acidic pharmaceuticals such as non-steroidal anti-inflammatory drugs and lipid regulators. Therefore, acid dissociation constants (pK_a) and pH are important parameters to understand the fate of acidic PhACs during soil passage.

2.4. Occurrence, fate and removal of bulk organic matter in managed aquifer recharge

2.4.1. Total organic carbon and dissolved organic carbon

During soil passage from source water to a production well, bulk organic matter is attenuated through physical, chemical and biological processes (i.e., filtration, sorption and biodegradation). The fate of bulk organic matter during soil passage can be characterized using a suite of both routine and innovative analytical tools. The most common method to quantify the amount of bulk organic matter is total organic carbon (TOC) or dissolved organic carbon (DOC). Moreover, subtracting DOC values of BF and AR filtrates from source water are often used to determine the removal of biodegradable organic carbon during soil passage. Generally, TOC and DOC removal efficiencies ranged from 30 to 88% and 33 to 88%, respectively (Table 2.1). The removal of TOC and DOC dominantly occurs within the first few meters of infiltration and is mainly due to biodegradation (i.e., biologically active colmation layer) (Hiscock and Grischek, 2002; Quanrud et al., 2003).

2.4.2. Specific UV absorbance

Specific UV absorbance (SUVA) is the ratio of DOC and UV absorbance at 254 nm and represents the relative aromaticity of organic matter (Amy and Drewes, 2007). SUVA was observed to increase from 2.1 L/m-mg to 2.4 L/m-mg during infiltration under oxic conditions at the Lake Tegel BF site (Berlin, Germany), and the increase of SUVA suggested a preferential removal of aliphatic organic matter during soil passage (Grünheid et al., 2005). At a BF site in Parkville (Missouri, USA), the average SUVA from the production wells was higher than that of the surface water (Missouri river) during a month of monitoring (Weiss et al., 2004). The Sweetwater recharge facilities located in Tucson (Arizona, USA) monitored SUVA during 1996-2001, and SUVA increased by 30-80% during infiltration through the first meter of infiltration basin sediments (Quanrud et al., 2003). Cha et al. (2004) and Maeng et al (2008) used river water and canal water, respectively, to investigate the fate of bulk organic matter during BF using columns. They also showed that SUVA values increased with travel distances and residence times. In contrast, SUVA values from BF sites in Jeffersonville and Terre Haute (USA) were highly varied, and there was no universal change for SUVA (Weiss et al., 2004). However, other NOM characterization tools described below have demonstrated the preferential removal of non-humic substances (i.e., aliphatic organic matter) during soil passage. Therefore, aliphatic organic matter is preferentially removed during BF and AR.

Table 2.1 Overview of TOC and DOC removal efficiencies in managed aquifer recharge systems worldwide

Site	Distance (meter)	Residence time (day)	Types	C_o (TOC/DOC) mg/L	TOC removal (%)	DOC removal (%)	Well Type	Capacity (m^3/s)	References
Hämeenlinna, Finland	1000-1300	90	AR[3]	14/	88		V[4]		(Kolehmainen et. al., 2007)
Jyväskylä, Finland	200-550	15-30	AR[3]	9/	77		V[4]		(Kolehmainen et. al., 2007)
Tuusula, Finland	500-700	30-60	AR[3]	6/	73		V[4]		(Kolehmainen et. al., 2007)
Louisville, Kentucky, USA	30.5	120	RBF[1]	2.9/	30	33	H[5]	0.88	(Wang et. al., 2002)
Jeffersonville, Indiana, USA	61	3-5	RBF[1]	3.0/2.7	60	58	V[4]	0.23	(Weiss et. al., 2004)
Jeffersonville, Indiana, USA	177	13-19	RBF[1]	3.0/2.7	75	74	V[4]	0.23	(Weiss et. al., 2004)
Terre Haute, Indiana, USA	27	13-19	RBF[1]	4.7/4.1	67	64	H[5]	0.53	(Weiss et. al., 2004)
Terre Haute, Indiana, USA	122	NA	RBF[1]	4.7/4.1	88	88	V[4]	0.044	(Weiss et. al., 2004)
Parkville, Missouri, USA	37	NA	RBF[1]	4.5/3.6	41	35	V[4]	0.075	(Weiss et. al., 2004)
Parkville, Missouri, USA	24	NA	RBF[1]	4.5/3.6	40	36	V[4]	0.075	(Weiss et. al., 2004)
Pembroke, New Hampshire, USA	55	5	RBF[1]	/1.5-7		71	V[4]		(Partinoudi and Collins, 2007)
Berlin (Lake Tegel), Germany	100	135	LBF[2]	/7.5		42	V[4]		(Grunheid et. al., 2005)
Berlin (Lake Tegel), Germany	77	117	LBF[2]	/7.2-7.5		34-40	V[4]		(Grunheid et. al., 2005)
Berlin (Lake Tegel), Germany	32	50	AR[3]	/7.2-7.5		34-40	V[4]		(Grunheid et. al., 2005)
Düsseldorf, Germany	50		RBF[1]	/4.3		40	H[5]		(Schubert, 2002)
Monitoring well-MW5, Tuscon, Arizona, USA	6	11	AR[3]	/14.1		66	V[4]		(Amy and Drewes, 2007)

[1] RBF: riverbank filtration; [2] LBF: lake bank filtration; [3] AR: artificial recharge; [4] V: vertical, [5] H: horizontal

Table 2.1 (continued)

Site	Distance (meter)	Residence time (day)	Types	C_o (TOC/DOC) mg/L	TOC removal (%)	DOC removal (%)	Well Type	Capacity (m^3/s)	References
Monitoring well WR199, Tuscon, Arizona, USA	35	35	AR3	/14.1		93	V4		(Amy and Drewes, 2007)
Monitoring well-NW4, Mesa, Arizona, USA	388	6-18 (month)	AR3	/6.10		76	V4		(Amy and Drewes, 2007)
Monitoring well-NW3, Mesa, Arizona, USA	655	6-19 (month)	AR3	/6.10		71	V4		(Amy and Drewes, 2007)
Monitoring well-NW2, Mesa, Arizona, USA	885	6-20 (month)	AR3	/6.10		75	V4		(Amy and Drewes, 2007)
Monitoring well-10U, Mesa, Arizona, USA	1950	12-96 (month)	AR3	/6.10		81	V4		(Amy and Drewes, 2007)
Monitoring well-26U, Mesa, Arizona, USA	1950	12-96 (month)	AR3	/6.10		88	V4		(Amy and Drewes, 2007)
Monitoring well-44U, Mesa, Arizona, USA	2700	12-96 (month)	AR3	/6.10		82	V4		(Amy and Drewes, 2007)

[1] RBF: riverbank filtration; [2] LBF: lake bank filtration; [3] AR: artificial recharge; [4] V: vertical, [5] H: horizontal

2.4.3. XAD Resin Fractionation

XAD-8 fractionation is often used to characterize NOM fractions for many applications, and the XAD-8 resin column separates NOM into hydrophobic and hydrophilic fractions of organic matter. Weiss et al. (2004) investigated the change in NOM fractions during RBF using XAD-8 columns, and suggested that there was no clear relationship in removal from different NOM fractions. Removal efficiencies of the hydrophilic fraction from three BF sites in the USA (Jeffersonville, Terre Haute, and Parkville) ranged between 40 and 70%, and removal efficiencies of hydrophobic fraction varied between 35 and 60% (Weiss et al., 2004). Rauch and Drewes (2004) found in column studies that hydrophilic organic matter in secondary effluent isolated using chromatographic resin (XAD-8) was removed to a higher degree compared to hydrophobic organic matter. Xue et al. (2009) used XAD-8/XAD-4 resin chromatography to fractionate five classes of NOM, and showed 80% of hydrophilic organic matter was removed by aerobic biodegradation. They found that hydrophilic organic matter exhibits the highest biodegradability compared to other four NOM fractions (e.g., hydrophobic acid, hydrophobic neutral, transphilic acid and transphilic neutral). During 5-year of program conducted at the Sweetwater recharge facilities (Tucson, Arizona, USA), hydrophilic organic matter was also preferentially removed during soil passage (Quanrud et al., 2003). Based on the results obtained using XAD-8 and/or XAD-4 resin chromatography, there was a preferential removal of hydrophilic organic matter during soil passage. Hydrophilic organic matter contains a relatively high amount of aliphatic organic matter (Rauch and Drewes, 2004), consistent with SUVA results discussed in the previous section; both approaches suggest that aliphatic organic matter was preferentially removed.

2.4.4. Size Exclusion Chromatography

A LC-OCD (Liquid Chromatography-Organic Carbon Detector) (i.e., size exclusion chromatography) system using a liquid chromatography method describes the molecular weight (MW) distribution and classification of organic matter according to biopolymers, humic substances, building blocks, neutrals and low MW acids. These fractions are quantified as organic carbon concentration using an organic carbon detector and characterized by a UV detector. More details of this system are described in Huber and Frimmel (1992). The major NOM fraction change during soil passage (Lake Tegel site, Berlin, Germany) was the biopolymer fraction which is the largest MW fraction (MW>20,000 Da) in a LC-OCD chromatogram, and is comprised of non-humic substances (Grünheid and Jekel, 2005; Jekel and Grünheid, 2005). Samples from the production well at the Lake Tegel BF site showed an almost complete removal of the biopolymer fraction, even at the first monitoring well from the lake. An AR site located at Lake Tegel, Berlin (Germany) treats the same lake water as the BF site but uses infiltration basins instead of extraction from the lake by a hydraulic gradient (Grünheid et al., 2005). Again, the biopolymer fraction was significantly removed, and other fractions were partially removed. Kolehmainen et al (2007) suggested that large MW fractions in the river water were more efficiently removed compared to the smaller fractions during AR. Thus, significant removal of the biopolymer fraction in infiltrated water was observed. The biopolymer fraction is comprised of easily biodegradable organic matter (i.e., non-humic) such as proteins and polysaccharides. The preferential removal of the biopolymer (non-humic) fraction corresponds to the increase of SUVA which was due to the removal of aliphatic organic matter during soil passage.

2.4.5. Fluorescence Excitation-Emission Matrices

Fluorescence Excitation (ex)-Emission (em) Matrices (F-EEM) provide fluorescence intensity (FI) peaks at known wavelengths of humic-like peaks P1 (ex/em=250-260/380-480 nm) and P2 (ex/em=330-350/420-480 nm) and a protein-like peak, P3 (ex/em=270-280/320-350 nm) (Leenheer and Croue, 2003). Several previous studies have demonstrated P1, P2 and P3 have been associated with humic-like and protein-like substances (Coble, 1996; Chen et al., 2003; Henderson et al., 2009). Column studies simulating BF showed that there was a preferential removal of protein-like substances compared to humic-like substances during infiltration (Maeng et al, 2008). Previous studies have also reported that significant amounts of protein-like substances were attenuated during soil passage using reclaimed wastewater (Amy and Drewes 2007; Xue 2009). These results also correspond to LC-OCD results from Lake Tegel that the biopolymer fraction (e.g., protein-like substances) was effectively removed by BF. On the basis of the results of SUVA, F-EEM and LC-OCD, it can be concluded that there is a preferential removal of non-humic substances during soil passage, and this removal was attributed to microbial activity.

2.4.6. Polarity Rapid Assessment Method

The polarity rapid assessment method (PRAM) characterizes the polarity of bulk organic matter by measuring the fraction of substances adsorbed onto different solid-phase extraction (SPE) sorbents (Rosario-Ortiz et al., 2004; Rosario-Ortiz et al., 2007a; Rosario-Ortiz et al., 2009). Non-polar sorbents (C18, C8 and C2), polar sorbents (CN, silica and diol) and anionic sorbents (NH2 and SAX) are commonly used to characterize the polarity of bulk organic matter under ambient conditions. Non-polar sorbents and polar sorbents extract hydrophobic organic matter and hydrophilic organic matter, respectively. Anionic sorbents extract negatively charged organic matter. PRAM uses the normalized UV absorbance breakthrough curve to determine the amount of total materials adsorbed, defined as a retention coefficient (RC). RC is expressed as $1-C_{max}/C_0$ (C_{max}: maximum absorbance after break through curve and C_0: absorbance of original sample) (Rosario-Ortiz et al., 2007b; Philibert et al., 2008). Using different properties of sorbents, PRAM analysis depicts different degrees of polarity in bulk organic matter originating from different sources or water treatment steps.

Since PRAM has been recently introduced, there are only few published data on its use in studies related to soil passage. PRAM was carried out in a study using soil columns (Maeng et al., 2008). Three different solvents, C18, silica and amino, were used for samples derived from column studies simulating BF. PRAM demonstrated that the non-polar character of organic matter (C18) (i.e., hydrophobic component) slightly decreased during infiltration using column studies simulating BF, with fractions in influent and effluent samples corresponding to 20 and 15%, respectively. Uncharged polar character (hydrophilic organic matter) significantly decreased during infiltration, corresponding to a reduction in biopolymer fraction (i.e., hydrophilic-neutral) from LC-OCD analysis, as explained above. The anionic fraction of NOM slightly increased after infiltration due to a reduction of neutral organic matter (i.e., aliphatic organic matter). PRAM can be used as an analytical tool and provides insightful information about variability in bulk organic matter characteristics during soil passage.

2.5. Occurrence, fate and removal of pharmaceutically active compounds in managed aquifer recharge

A summary of a literature review on removal efficiencies of 9 different categories of PhACs, based on therapeutic uses, during BF or AR is presented in Table 2.2 Each BF/AR site was analyzed with respect to well types, travel distances, residence times and redox conditions. Detail information of site characteristics are presented in Table 2.3.

2.5.1. Antibiotics

The occurrence and fate of antibiotics in the aquatic environment is of growing interest, but only a few studies have been carried out to investigate their fate during BF and AR. Heberer et al. (2008) investigated 19 targeted antibiotics at a lake BF site located in Berlin (Germany) for 2.5 years. This site is well characterized and instrumented in terms of both production wells and transects of monitoring wells where travel distances, residence times, and redox conditions are defined. They detected 7 out of 19 target antibiotics in Lake Wannsee water used for BF: sulfamethoxazole, acetyl-sulfamethoxazole, anhydroerythromycin, clarithromycin, roxithromycin, trimethoprim and clindamycin. However, all antibiotics were completely removed after less than 2-4 months of travel times except for sulfamethoxazole. Sulfamethoxazole was detected at the production well, but it was present at a very low concentration (2 ng/L) compared to the concentration found in Lake Wannsee (155 ng/L). From the results of several monitoring wells installed along the transect, Heberer et al. (2008) suggested that sulfamethoxazole was more efficiently removed under anoxic conditions (~99%) than under oxic conditions (~52%).

Grünheid et al. (2005) compared bulk organic matter and organic micropollutant removal between BF and AR sites located in Berlin (Germany). This BF site exhibited oxic conditions followed by prolonged anoxic conditions, whereas the AR mainly showed oxic conditions. The removal of sulfamethoxazole at the BF site was relatively higher (75%) than that at the AR site (50%). However, Heberer et al. (2008) suggested that it was not possible to determine if redox conditions control the degradation of sulfamethoxazole in the study done by Grünheid et al. (2005) because of the different residence times between the BF site and the AR site. Longer residence times at the BF site could also lead to a better removal of sulfamethoxazole. Schmidt et al. (2007) also investigated sulfamethoxazole, clarithromycin, trimethoprim and clindamycin at four BF sites located along the river Rhine (Rhine A and Rhine B), Elbe and Ruhr. They also found that selected antibiotics were removed greater than >70% except sulfamethoxazole which exhibited relatively low removal (0-25%) at Rhine A and Rhine B sites (mainly oxic conditions). However, greater than 90% removal efficiencies of sulfamethoxazole were achieved at Ruhr BF site which has relatively short residence times compared to Rhine A and Rhine B but mainly exhibits anaerobic conditions. This study supports the results from Grünheid et al. (2005) that sulfamethoxazole is a redox dependent compound which degrades more effectively under anoxic/anaerobic conditions. From the results described above it can be concluded that MAR is an effective treatment step in a multi-barrier system of drinking water supply for antibiotic removal.

2.5.2. Non-steroidal anti-inflammatory drug (NSAID) and

analgesics

NSAIDs, also known as pain killers, are commonly used for symptoms of arthritis, bursitis, gout, swelling, stiffness and joint pain around the world (Metcalfe et al., 2004). Large amounts of NSAIDs are sold by prescription or non-prescription worldwide (i.e., over the counter drugs) (Heberer, 2002). High concentrations of NSAIDs have been detected in aquatic environments and wastewater due to their high consumption in human medical care and, to some degree, because of their persistent characteristics (Zhou et al., 2009). Many NSAIDs mentioned in this paper have been removed to greater than 50% during BF and AR. A number of field and laboratory-scale studies have shown significant removals of diclofenac, ibuprofen, naproxen and phenazone during soil passage (Heberer and Adam, 2004; Massmann et al., 2006; Schmidt et al., 2007; Snyder et al., 2007; Massmann et al., 2008). Biodegradation or biotransformation (biotic) and sorption (abiotic) are possible mechanisms for NSAIDs removal. Diclofenac, ibuprofen, indomethacin and naproxen have moderately high octanol-water partition coefficients (log $K_{ow} > 2.5$), and adsorption would likely be the main mechanism of their removal during soil passage. However, several studies demonstrated biodegradation potentials of some NSAIDs in laboratory-scale experiments (Kagle et al., 2009). For example, ibuprofen was biologically transformed in microcosms prepared with sediment and fortified lake water (Buser et al., 1999; Lin et al., 2006). Transformation products (e.g., carboxyibuprofen and hydroxyibuprofen) were detected in a cultivated river water reactor, confirming partial biodegradation of ibuprofen (Winkler et al., 2001). The majority of NSAIDs are acidic compounds that exist as ionic species during soil passage, with pK_a values of many NSAIDs being lower than the pH of aquatic environments (e.g., diclofenac pK_a 4.2, ibuprofen pK_a 4.9, and naproxen pK_a 4.2). KOWWIN^{TM} was used to estimate log K_{ow} (USEPA, 2009), and naproxen exhibits 3.18 for log K_{ow} which shows moderate hydrophobicity. However, naproxen predominantly exists as an ionized form in the aqueous phase because of its low pK_a (4.2). The log D (distribution coefficient at pH 8) of naproxen is 0.53, suggesting ionic interactions may have more influence on the removal of naproxen than adsorption during soil passage. Therefore, pH is an important parameter to investigate the fate of acidic compounds, and log D (instead of log K_{ow}) should be used for acidic PhACs such as NSAIDs to indicate their characteristics (Cunningham, 2004).

Phenazone-type pharmaceuticals, another type of NSAIDs, are redox dependent compounds that are removed to a higher degree under oxic conditions than under anoxic conditions. According to Massmann et al. (2006), the removal of phenazone at an AR site varied by season and was relatively high during winter compared to summer. This was due to oxic conditions that mainly occurred at the AR site during winter when temperatures were low. Moreover, the AR site also showed higher removal efficiencies for phenazone-type pharmaceuticals including phenazone (91%), propyphenazone (100%) and DMAA (Dimethylaminophenazone) metabolites such as formylaminoantipyrine (FAA) (89%) and acetoaminoantipyrine (AAA) (96%). However, AMDOPH, which is another DMAA metabolite, was almost persistent under all conditions (removal <5%). Massmann et al. (2008) found similar results at a BF site located at Lake Wannsee (Berlin, Germany) using two monitoring wells installed between Lake Wannsee and the production well. The removal of phenazone (66%) in an oxic monitoring well was relatively high, whereas the phenazone removal in an anoxic monitoring well was very low (10%). Their study confirms that there is a preferential removal of phenazone-type pharmaceuticals under oxic conditions. Massmann et al. (2006) suggested that biodegradation by aerobic bacteria was the main removal mechanism of phenazone-type pharmaceuticals during soil passage. Based on previous studies described above, it is important to monitor pH during soil passage because many of NSAIDs remain as ionic species in the aquatic environment. Moreover, some NSAIDs (e.g., phenazone-type pharmaceuticals) are redox dependent; thus, it is equally important to monitor redox conditions during BF and AR.

2.5.3. Anticonvulsants

Anticonvulsant pharmaceuticals are the most persistent type during BF and AR. Among the anticonvulsants, there have been many studies carried out on carbamazepine because it is the most frequently detected anticonvulsants in the environment (Drewes et al., 2002; Heberer et al., 2002; Cordy et al., 2004; Heberer and Adam, 2004; Mechlinski and Heberer, 2005; Massmann et al., 2006; Schmidt et al., 2007). Carbamazepine has shown a persistent behavior in the aquatic environment, and the poor biodegradability of carbamazepine results in low removal (<10%) in most wastewater treatment plants (Ternes, 1998; Stamatelatou et al., 2003; Zhang et al., 2008; Kasprzyk-Hordern et al., 2009). Moreover, Clara et al. (2004) proposed carbamazepine as a marker for anthropogenic influences in the aquatic environment. A number of laboratory and field studies on BF and AR have also revealed low removals of primidone and dilantin during infiltration (Heberer and Adam, 2004; Heberer et al., 2004). Drewes et al. (2002) found that there was no change in carbamazepine and primidone concentrations during soil aquifer treatment for estimated travel times of up to 6 years. Based on the performance of selected anticonvulsants in these studies, BF and AR are not effective in the removal of anticonvulsants.

2.5.4. Antidepressants

Three antidepressants (fluoxetine, meprobamate and diazepam) were chosen by Snyder et al. (2007) to investigate their fate during BF using a pilot plant. Among the studied antidepressants, fluoxetine was found to be removed significantly (>99%) and average removal efficiencies observed in column studies for meprobamate and diazepam were 66% and 36%, respectively. A higher removal of fluoxetine can be attributed mainly to adsorption based on its high octanol water partition coefficient (log K_{ow}: 4.69). Due to limited information and studies done on antidepressants during subsurface infiltration, it is not possible to characterize the performance of BF and AR in antidepressant removals.

2.5.5. Beta blockers

According to Schmidt et al. (2007), four beta blockers (atenolol, metoprolol, bisoprolol and sotalol) were removed greater than 70% at BF sites located along the rivers Rhine, Elbe and Ruhr. Five beta blockers; atenolol (0.36 µg/L), sotalol (1.3 µg/L), celiprolol (0.28 µg/L), propranolol (0.18 µg/L) and metoprolol (1.7 µg/L); in secondary effluent were found to be below the limit of quantification (0.025 µg/L) after soil aquifer treatment using agricultural fields in Braunschweig, (Germany) (Ternes et al., 2007). This study suggested that selected beta blockers were removed by sorption and/or biodegradation during soil passage. In contrast, in some recent studies, low removals of beta blockers were observed during wastewater treatment processes (Castiglioni et al., 2005; Kasprzyk-Hordern et al., 2009; Wick et al., 2009). As a consequence, beta blockers are often detected in the aquatic environment in the ng/L to µg/L range (Wick et al., 2009). Further study is required to understand the removal of beta blockers observed during subsurface infiltration compared to wastewater treatment processes.

2.5.6. Lipid regulators

Like NSAIDs, many lipid regulators remain as ionic species in the aquatic environment (Mompelat et al. 2009). Thus, pH during subsurface infiltration plays an important role in the removal mechanism of lipid regulators. Metabolites of lipid regulators (e.g., clofibric acid and fenofibric acid) are important to monitor during soil passage because they are derived from "prodrugs", administered in an inactive form. A prodrug undergoes metabolic conversion of the parent compound to an active metabolite which cures the symptoms, not the parent compound which is an inactive form (e.g., clofibrate and fenofibrate). Clofibric acid, fenofibric acid and salicylic acid are common metabolites originating from clofibrate, fenofibrate and aspirin, respectively. Clofibric acid is one of the most common metabolites studied for BF and AR, and it is often detected in the aquatic environment, wetlands and wastewater treatment plants (Winkler et al., 2001; Heberer, 2002; Matamoros et al., 2008; Dordio et al., 2009; Kagle et al., 2009). According to Heberer et al. (2004), clofibric acid concentrations increased at the production wells located at the Lake Tegel BF site, Berlin (Germany). This was due to a high consumption of the fibrate-based lipid regulators during the 1990s. The use of fibrate-based lipid regulators has been significantly reduced over the last 10 years, but clofibric acid still remains in deeper layers of the aquifer (Heberer et al. 2004). Therefore, "old" bank filtrate still exhibits a high concentration of clofibric acid from the 1990's. However, BF sites along the river Rhine and an AR site located at Lake Tegel removed clofibric acid greater than 70% (Heberer and Adam, 2004; Heberer et al., 2004; Schmidt et al., 2007). Moreover, bezafibrate was found to be significantly removed during subsurface infiltration (Heberer, 2002). Thus, the removal performance of lipid regulators in BF and AR systems varied from site to site.

2.5.7. X-Ray contrast media

Grünheid et al. (2005) conducted field studies at BF and AR sites (Lake Tegel, Berlin, Germany). to investigate the fate of X-ray contrast agents which can be measured as adsorbable organic iodine (AOI) Redox conditions at the BF site gradually changed from oxic to prolonged anoxic conditions along the flow pathway, but at the AR site, mainly the oxic conditions prevailed. Both the BF and AR sites used water from Lake Tegel for infiltration. AOI removal efficiencies at the BF site and the AR sites were 60% and 30%, respectively. The removal efficiency of AOI at the BF site was higher than that at the AR site. Grünheid et al. (2005) found that AOI removal efficiencies and ORP (oxidation-reduction potential) were inversely correlated, and dehalogenation of AOI was enhanced under anoxic conditions. They also showed that AOI concentrations changed by season in infiltrated water as a result of the discharge of wastewater effluent into the lake; this was due to variations of dilution in wastewater effluent discharges. Schittko et al. (2004) obtained similar results at the same BF site, where 63% of AOI was removed during soil passage. Beside AOI, four individual iodinated X-ray contrast agents (iopromide, iopamidol, iomeprol and ioxhexol) were measured at different BF sites located in Germany (Schittko et al., 2004; Grünheid et al., 2005; Schmidt et al., 2007). Iopromide, iopamidol and iomeprol were significantly removed (>80%) and found to be easily removable compounds during BF.

2.5.8. Steroid hormones

Steroid hormones such as synthetic estrogens (e.g., 17α-ethinylestradiol) and natural estrogens (e.g., estrone and 17β-estradiol) are of special concern because of potential adverse effects on human health and aquatic life at very low concentration (<5ng/L) (Mansell and Drewes, 2004a). A number of laboratory-scale and field studies on the fate of estrogens during soil passage have been carried out (Mansell and Drewes 2004a, Mansell et al. 2004b; Snyder et al. 2004; Zuehlke et al. 2004). A field study carried out by Zuehlke et al. (2004) showed that 17β-estradiol (E2) and 17α-ethinylestradiol (EE2) were not detected in the surface water from Berlin (LOQ: 0.2 ng/L), and estrone (E1) was removed greater than 80% at a monitoring well located close to the lake shore. This study demonstrated that a significant removal of E1 was possible during soil passage even within a short distance . Estrogen compounds are generally hydrophobic compounds which are typically neutral; thus, adsorption is likely to be the main removal mechanism. Mansell and Drewes (2004a) performed field studies combined with laboratory-scale experiments and showed that estriol (E3) and testosterone were significantly removed to below their detection limits (E3: < 0.6 ng/L, testosterone: < 0.5 ng/L). Their study also suggested that biodegradation increased removal efficiencies of E1, E2 and EE2. Snyder et al. (2004) also showed similar results using batch experiments and field studies, and demonstrated biodegradation and significant attenuation of estrogen compounds (e.g., E1, E2, EE2 and testosterone). Mansell et al. (2004b) also found that steroids were removed below the detection limit by a combination of adsorption and biodegradation; thus, the removal of estrogen compounds is not only dependent on adsorption, but is also affected by biodegradation. Ying et al. (2003) conducted an experiment with E2 in aquifer materials using groundwater, and found that E2 was rapidly degraded in aquifer materials under aerobic conditions but remained almost unchanged under anaerobic conditions. This study suggested that the removal of E2 can be enhanced by aerobic bacteria and was not observed under anaerobic conditions. Thus, aerobic bacteria also play an important role in the removal of E2. Based on the studies mentioned above, it can be concluded that MAR is an effective and reliable treatment for removing estrogenic compounds.

Table 2.2 Removal efficiencies of different class of pharmaceutically active compounds during managed aquifer recharge treatment

Therapeutic use	Compound	Removal efficiencies (%)				References
		Low (<25%)	Moderately low (26-50)	Relatively high (51-79)	High (>80)	
Antibiotics	Sulfamethoxazole	Rhine A (0-25), Rhine B (0-25), Lake Tegel-LBF[27] (8)	Lake Wannsee[13] (46), Lake Tegel-AR[5] (35), Lake Tegel-AR[6] (42)	Lake Tegel-AR[1] (75), Lake Tegel-AR[7] (53), Elbe (>70), Lake Wannsee[15] (64), Lake Wannsee[16] (62), Lake Wannsee[19] (52), Lake Wannsee[20] (75), Lake Wannsee[21] (72), Column[5](65), Lake Tegel-LBF[14] (63), Lake Tegel-LBF[16] (54), Lake Tegel-LBF[18] (69), Lake Tegel-LBF[31] (70)	Lake Wannsee[3] (99), Lake Tegel-LBF[1] (95), Ruhr(>80), Lake Wannsee[14] (97), Lake Wannsee[17] (96), Lake Wannsee[18] (99), Column[4](95), Lake Tegel-LBF[15] (91), Lake Tegel-LBF[17] (85), Lake Tegel-LBF[20] (83), Lake Tegel-LBF[19] (83), Lake Tegel-LBF[21] (98), Lake Tegel-LBF[1] (95), Lake Tegel-LBF[29] (82), Lake Tegel-LBF[31] (80)	Grünheid et al. (2005), Schmidt et al. (2007), Heberer et al. (2008), Grünheid and Jekel (2005), Jekel and Grünheid (2005)
	Acetyl-sulfamethoxazole				Lake Wannsee[3] (>90), Lake Wannsee[18] (>99), Lake Wannsee[19] (>99), Lake Wannsee[20] (>99), Lake Wannsee[21] (>99)	Heberer et al. (2008)
	Clarithromycin			Rhine A (>70), Elbe (>70), Ruhr (>70)	Lake Wannsee[3] (>90), Lake Wannsee[18] (>90), Lake Wannsee[19] (>90), Lake Wannsee[20] (>90), Lake Wannsee[21] (>90)	Schmidt et al. (2007), Heberer et al. (2008)
	Roxithromycin			Ruhr (>70)	Lake Wannsee[3] (>90), Lake Wannsee[18] (>98), Lake Wannsee[19] (>90), Lake Wannsee[20] (>90), Lake Wannsee[21] (>90)	Schmidt et al. (2007), Heberer et al. (2008)
	Trimethoprim				Lake Wannsee[3] (>90), Lake Wannsee[18] (>92), Lake Wannsee[19] (>92), Lake Wannsee[20] (>92), Lake Wannsee[21] (>92), Rhine A (>80), Elbe (>80), Ruhr (>80)	Heberer et al. (2008), Schmidt et al. (2007)
	Clindamycin		Lake Wannsee[18] (26)	Rhine B (>70), Elbe (>70), Ruhr (>70)	Lake Wannsee[3] (>98), Lake Wannsee[19] (93), Lake Wannsee[20] (>99.68), Lake Wannsee[21] (>99.68), Rhine A (>80)	Heberer et al. (2008), Schmidt et al. (2007)
Antidepressants	Meprobamate			Column 1 (53), Column 2 (71), Column 3 (74)		Snyder et al. (2007)
	Fluoxetine				Column 1 (>99), Column 2 (>99), Column 3 (>99)	Snyder et al. (2007)
	Diazepam	Column 1 (-8)	Column 2 (42)	Column 2 (65)		Snyder et al. (2007)

Table 2.2 (continued)

Therapeutic use	Compound	Removal efficiencies (%) Low (<25%)	Moderately low (26-50)	Relatively high (51-79)	High (>80)	References
Non-steroidal anti-inflammatory drugs (NSAIDs) and analgesics	Diclofenac			Column 1 (67), Lake Wannsee[4] (60), Lake Tegel-LBF[13](>67)	Rhine A (>80), Rhine B (>80), Elbe (>80), Ruhr (>80), Lake Tegel-AR[3] (93), Column 2(>99), Column 3 (>99), Lake Wannsee[5] (>80), Lake Wannsee[6] (80), Lake Wannsee[12] (>81), Lake Wannsee[24] (80), Lake Wannsee[25] (>93), Lake Wannsee[26] (87)	Heberer and Adam (2004), Snyder et al. (2007), Schmidt et al. (2007), Heberer et al. (2004)
	Ibuprofen				Rhine A (>80), Elbe (>80), Ruhr (>80), Column 1 (>99), Column 2(>99), Column 3 (>99)	Schmidt et al. (2007), Snyder et al. (2007)
	Indomethacin			Rhine A (>70), Elbe (>70), Lake Wannsee[8] (>71)	Lake Tegel-AR[3] (>95), Lake Wannsee-well[4] (>99), Lake Wannsee-well[5] (>99), Lake Wannsee-well[6] (>99), Lake Wannsee[9] (>94), Lake Wannsee[10] (>94), Lake Wannsee[11] (>94), Lake Wannsee[12] (>94), Lake Wannsee[24](>93), Lake Wannsee[25] (>93), Lake Wannsee[26] (>93)	Schmidt et al. (2007), Heberer and Adam (2004), Heberer et al. (2004), Heberer et al..(2003b) & Pekdeger (2006), Heberer et al.(2003a)
	Naproxen			Elbe (>70), Ruhr (>70)	Rhine A (>80), Column 1 (>98), Column 2 (>98), Column 3 (>98)	Schmidt et al. (2007), Snyder et al. (2007)
	Phenazone	Lake Wannsee[2] (10)		Lake Wannsee[1] (66)	Lake Tegel-AR[4] (91)	Massmann et al. (2006), Massmann et al. (2008)
	FAA (formylaminoantipyrine)		Lake Wannsee[2] (36)	Lake Wannsee[1] (72)	Lake Tegel-AR[4] (89)	Massmann et al. (2006), Massmann et al. (2008)
	AAA (acetoaminoantipyrine)		Lake Wannsee[2] (45)		Lake Wannsee[1] (90), Lake Tegel-AR[4] (96)	Massmann et al. (2006), Massmann et al. (2008)
	AMDOPH (1-acetyl-1-methyl-2-dimethyloxamoyl-2-phenylhydrazide)	Lake Wannsee[1] (0), Lake Wannsee[2] (0), Lake Tegel-AR[4] (0)				Massmann et al. (2006), Massmann et al. (2008)
	Pentoxifyline				Rhine A (>80), Elbe (>80)	Schmidt et al. (2007)

32

Table 2.2 (continued)

Therapeutic use	Compound	Removal efficiencies (%)				References
		Low (<25%)	Moderately low (26-50)	Relatively high (51-79)	High (>80)	
Anticonvulsants	Carbamazepine	Rhine A (0-25), Rhine B (0-25), Lake Tegel-AR[4] (0), Column 1 (-3), Column 2 (22), Column 3 (13), Lake Tegel-LBF[9] (15), Lake Wannsee[7] (10)		Elbe (51-70)	Ruhr (>80)	Massmann et al. (2006), Schmidt et al. (2007), Snyder et al. (2007), Mechlinski and Heberer (2005)
	Dilantin	Column 1 (-11), Column 3 (22)	Column 2 (28)			Snyder et al. (2007)
	Primidone	Tucson (0), Lake Wannsee[8] (-11), Lake Wannsee[9] (-2), Lake Wannsee[10] (18), Lake Wannsee[11] (5)	Lake Wannsee[4] (33), Lake Wannsee[6] (42), Lake Tegel-AR[3] (26), Lake Wannsee[24] (45), Lake Wannsee[26] (45)		Lake Wannsee-well[5] (83)	Heberer and Adam (2004), Heberer et al. (2004) Drewes et al. (2002), Heberer et al. (2003b) & Pekdeger (2006), Heberer et al.(2003a)
Beta blockers	Atenolol				Rhine A (>80), Elbe (>80), Ruhr (>80)	Schmidt et al. (2007)
	Metoprolol,				Rhine A (>80), Rhine B (>80), Elbe (>80), Ruhr (>80)	Schmidt et al. (2007)
	Bisoprolol			Rhine A (>70), Ruhr (>70)		Schmidt et al. (2007)
	Sotalol				Rhine A (>80), Rhine B (>80), Elbe (>80), Ruhr (>80)	Schmidt et al. (2007)
Lipid regulators	Bezafibrate			Lake Tegel-LBF[13] (>75)	Rhine A (>80), Rhine B (>80), Elbe (>80), Ruhr (>80), Lake Tegel-AR[3] (>97), Lake Wannsee[8] (95%), Lake Wannsee[10] (>98), Lake Wannsee[9] (>98), Lake Wannsee[11] (>98), Lake Wannsee[12] (>98), Lake Wannsee[4] (>98), Lake Wannsee[5] (>98), Lake Wannsee[6] (>98), Lake Tegel-LBF[11] (>95), Lake Tegel-LBF[12] (>95)	Heberer and Adam (2004), Schmidt et al. (2007), Heberer et al. (2003b) & Pekdeger (2006), Heberer et al. (2004)

Table 2.2 (continued)

Therapeutic use	Compound	Removal efficiencies (%)				References
		Low (<25%)	Moderately low (26-50)	Relatively high (51-79)	High (>80)	
Lipid regulators	Fenofibric acid			Rhine A (>70), Rhine B (>70)		Schmidt et al. (2007)
	Clofibric acid	Lake Tegel-LBF[3](-20), Lake Wannsee[4] (-58), Lake Wannsee[5] (-92), Lake Wannsee[6] (-108), Lake Wannsee[12](-85), Lake Tegel-LBF[12](13), Lake Tegel-LBF[13](-25), Lake Tegel-LBF[33](-26), Lake Tegel-LBF[34](-53)		Lake Tegel-AR[3] (75), Lake Tegel-LBF[4](63), Lake Tegel-LBF[5](75), Lake Wannsee[8] (62), Lake Wannsee[9] (64), Lake Wannsee[10] (75), Lake Tegel-LBF[35](63,64,63), Lake Tegel-LBF[36](75,75,53), Lake Tegel-LBF[37](58,71)	Ruhr (>80), Lake Tegel-LBF[11](88), Lake Tegel-LBF[0](95), Lake Wannsee[11] (92), Lake Tegel-LBF[32](88,86,89), Lake Tegel-LBF[33](>99, >93), Lake Tegel-LBF[34] (>99, >99), Lake Tegel-LBF[37] (95),	Heberer and Adam (2004), Heberer et al. (2004), Schmidt et al. (2007), Scheytt et al. (2004), Heberer et al.(2003b) & Pekdeger (2006), Verstraeten et al.(2002)
	Gemfibrozil				Column 1 (>99), Column 2 (>99), Column 3 (>99)	Snyder et al. (2007)
X-ray contrast media	AOI		Lake Tegel-AR[1] (30)	Lake Tegel-LBF[1] (60), Lake Tegel-LBF[7] (63)		Grünheid et al. (2005) Schittko et al. (2004)
	Iopromide			Column 1 (64), Lake Tegel-LBF[8] (75), Wannsee[13] (65)	Lake Tegel-LBF[1] (98), Lake Tegel-LBF[7] (95), Lake Tegel-LBF[27] (82), Lake Tegel-LBF[28](97), Lake Tegel-LBF[29] (96), Lake Tegel-LBF[30] (98), Lake Tegel-LBF[31] (99), Lake Tegel-AR[1] (99), Lake Tegel-AR[5] (89), Lake Tegel-AR[6] (98), Lake Tegel-AR[7] (99), Rhine A (98), Rhine B (>80), Elbe (>80), Ruhr (>80), Column 2(93), Column 3 (95), Lake Wannsee[14] (97), Lake Wannsee[15] (99), Lake Wannsee[16] (99), Wannsee[17] (98)	Grünheid et al. (2005) Schmidt et al. (2007) Snyder et al. (2007) Schittko et al. (2004), Grünheid and Jekel (2005)
	Iopamidol	Rhine A (0-25)			Ruhr (>80)	Schmidt et al. (2007)
	Iomeprol		Rhine B (26-50)	Elbe (>70)	Rhine A (>80), Rhine B (>80), Elbe (>80), Ruhr (>80)	Schmidt et al. (2007)
	Ioxhexol				Rhine A (>80), Rhine B (>80), Elbe (>80), Ruhr (>80)	Schmidt et al. (2007)
	Diatrizoate			Lake Tegel-LBF[7] (69), Lake Tegel-LBF[8] (52)	Lake Tegel-LBF[10] (83)	Schittko et al. (2004)

34

Table 2.2 (continued)

Therapeutic use	Compound	Removal efficiencies (%)				References
		Low (<25%)	Moderately low (26-50)	Relatively high (51-79)	High (>80)	
Psycho stimulants	Caffeine				Column 1 (95), Column 2(97), Column 3 (98)	Snyder et al. (2007)
Steroid hormones	Estradiol (E2)				Column 1 (>99), Column 2 (>99), Column 3 (>99), NW2 (>99), NW4(>99), 2U(>99%), 6U(>99%)	Mansell and Drewes (2004a), Snyder et al. (2007)
	Estriol (E3)				Column 1 (>99), Column 2 (>99), Column 3 (>99), NW2 (>99), NW4(>99), 2U(>99%), 6U(>99%)	Mansell and Drewes (2004a), Snyder et al. (2007)
	Estrone (E1)				Lake Tegel-LBF[2] (>99), Lake Tegel-AR[2] (>99), Column 1 (>99), Column 2 (>99), Column 3 (>99)	Zuehlke et al. (2004), Snyder et al. (2007)
	Progesterone,				Column 1 (>99), Column 2 (>99), Column 3 (>99)	Snyder et al. (2007)
	Testosterone				Column 1 (>99), Column 2 (>99), Column 3 (>99), NW2 (>99), NW4(>99), 2U(>99%), 6U(>99%)	Mansell and Drewes (2004a), Snyder et al. (2007)

Table 2.3 Well types, travel distances, residence times, redox conditions for BF and AR sites described in Table 2.2

Name	Type	Source/well	Distance (meter)	Residence time (day)	Redox conditions	References
Lake Tegel-LBF[1]	LBF	Lake Tegel/13[+]	90	135	Anoxic	Grünheid et al. (2005)
Lake Tegel-LBF[2]	LBF	Lake Tegel/3301[++]	40	90	Anoxic	Zuehlke et al. 2004
Lake Tegel-LBF[3]	LBF	Lake Tegel/3301[++]	40	90	Anoxic	Heberer et al. (2004)
Lake Tegel-LBF[4]	LBF	Lake Tegel/12[+]	90	135	Anoxic	Scheytt et al. (2004)
Lake Tegel-LBF[5]	LBF	Lake Tegel/13[+]	90	135	Anoxic	Scheytt et al. (2004)
Lake Tegel-LBF[6]	LBF	Lake Tegel/14[+]	90	135	Anoxic	Scheytt et al. (2004)
Lake Tegel-LBF[7]	LBF	Lake Tegel/3301[++]	40	90	Anoxic	Schittko et al. (2004)
Lake Tegel-LBF[8]	LBF	Lake Tegel/3311[++]	0	<1	Oxic	Schittko et al. (2004)
Lake Tegel-LBF[9]	LBF	Lake Tegel/3311[++]	0	<1	Oxic	Mechlinski and Heberer (2005)
Lake Tegel-LBF[10]	LBF	Lake Tegel/13[+]	90	135	Anoxic	Schittko et al. (2004)
Lake Tegel-LBF[11]	LBF	Lake Tegel/3311[++]	0	<1	Oxic	Heberer et al. (2004)
Lake Tegel-LBF[12]	LBF	Lake Tegel/3301[++]	40	90	Anoxic	Heberer et al. (2004)
Lake Tegel-LBF[13]	LBF	Lake Tegel/13[+]	90	135	Anoxic	Heberer et al. (2004)
Lake Tegel-LBF[14]	LBF	Lake Tegel/3301[++]	40	90	Oxic	Jekel and Grünheid (2005)
Lake Tegel-LBF[15]	LBF	Lake Tegel/3301[++]	40	90	Anoxic	Jekel and Grünheid (2005)
Lake Tegel-LBF[16]	LBF	Lake Tegel/3302[++]	70	90	Oxic	Jekel and Grünheid (2005)
Lake Tegel-LBF[17]	LBF	Lake Tegel/3302[++]	70	90	Anoxic	Jekel and Grünheid (2005)
Lake Tegel-LBF[18]	LBF	Lake Tegel/3303[++]	95	117	Oxic	Jekel and Grünheid (2005)
Lake Tegel-LBF[19]	LBF	Lake Tegel/3303[++]	95	117	Anoxic	Jekel and Grünheid (2005)
Lake Tegel-LBF[20]	LBF	Lake Tegel/13[+]	90	135	Oxic	Jekel and Grünheid (2005)
Lake Tegel-LBF[21]	LBF	Lake Tegel/13[+]	90	135	Anoxic	Jekel and Grünheid (2005)
Lake Tegel-LBF[22]	LBF	Lake Tegel/3310[++]	2	<1	Oxic	Mechlinski and Heberer (2005)
Lake Tegel-LBF[23]	LBF	Lake Tegel/3301[++]	25	90	Anoxic	Mechlinski and Heberer (2005)
Lake Tegel-LBF[24]	LBF	Lake Tegel/3302[++]	55	90	Anoxic	Mechlinski and Heberer (2005)
Lake Tegel-LBF[25]	LBF	Lake Tegel/3303[++]	77	117	Anoxic	Mechlinski and Heberer (2005)
Lake Tegel-LBF[26]	LBF	Lake Tegel/13[+]	90	135	Anoxic	Mechlinski and Heberer (2005)
Lake Tegel-LBF[27]	LBF	Lake Tegel/3310[++]	2	<1	Oxic	Grünheid et al. (2005)
Lake Tegel-LBF[28]	LBF	Lake Tegel/371UP[++]	30	84	Anoxic	Grünheid et al. (2005)
Lake Tegel-LBF[29]	LBF	Lake Tegel/3301[++]	25	90	Anoxic	Grünheid et al. (2005)
Lake Tegel-LBF[30]	LBF	Lake Tegel/3302[++]	55	90	Anoxic	Grünheid et al. (2005)

Table 2.3 (continued)

Name	Type	Source/well	Distance (meter)	Residence time (day)	Redox conditions	References
Lake Tegel-LBF[31]	LBF	Lake Tegel/3303[++]	77	117	Anoxic	Grünheid et al. (2005)
Lake Tegel-LBF[32]	LBF	Lake Tegel/3301[++]	25	90	Anoxic	Verstraeten et al.(2002b)
Lake Tegel-LBF[33]	LBF	Lake Tegel/3302[++]	55	90	Anoxic	Verstraeten et al.(2002b)
Lake Tegel-LBF[34]	LBF	Lake Tegel/3303[++]	77	117	Anoxic	Verstraeten et al.(2002b)
Lake Tegel-LBF[35]	LBF	Lake Tegel/12[+]	90	135	Anoxic	Verstraeten et al.(2002b)
Lake Tegel-LBF[36]	LBF	Lake Tegel/13[+]	90	135	Anoxic	Verstraeten et al.(2002b)
Lake Tegel-LBF[37]	LBF	Lake Tegel/14[+]	90	135	Anoxic	Verstraeten et al.(2002b)
Lake Tegel-AR[1]	AR	Lake Tegel/well20[+]	50	50	Oxic	Grünheid et al. (2005)
Lake Tegel-AR[2]	AR	Lake Tegel/[7]	90	50	Oxic	Zuehlke et al. (2004)
Lake Tegel-AR[3]	AR	Lake Tegel/[7]	90	50	Oxic	Heberer and Adam (2004)
Lake Tegel-AR[4]	AR	Lake Tegel/TEG365[++]	<10	<3	Oxic	Massmann et al. (2006)
Lake Tegel-AR[5]	AR	Lake Tegel/365[++]	2	4	Oxic	Grünheid et al. (2005)
Lake Tegel-AR[6]	AR	Lake Tegel/368UP[++]	10	25	Oxic	Grünheid et al. (2005)
Lake Tegel-AR[7]	AR	Lake Tegel/369UP[++]	32	50	Oxic	Grünheid et al. (2005)
Lake Wannsee1	LBF	Lake Wannsee /BE206++	1.5	<30	Oxic	Massmann et al. (2008)
Lake Wannsee2	LBF	Lake Wannsee /BE205++	20	~30	Anoxic	Massmann et al. (2008)
Lake Wannsee3	LBF	Lake Wannsee /well#3+	75	>120	Anoxic	Heberer et al. (2008)
Lake Wannsee4	LBF	Lake Wannsee /well#3+	75	>120	Anoxic	Heberer et al. (2004)
Lake Wannsee5	LBF	Lake Wannsee /well#4+	100	>120	Anoxic	Heberer et al. (2004)
Lake Wannsee6	LBF	Lake Wannsee /well#5+		>120	Anoxic	Heberer et al. (2004)
Lake Wannsee7	LBF	Lake Wannsee /BE206++	1.5	<30	Oxic	Mechlinski and Heberer (2005)
Lake Wannsee8	LBF	Lake Wannsee /3339++	40	65	Oxic	Heberer et al.,(2003b) & Pekdeger (2006)
Lake Wannsee9	LBF	Lake Wannsee /3338++	10	30	Oxic	Heberer et al.,(2003b) & Pekdeger (2006)
Lake Wannsee10	LBF	Lake Wannsee /3337++	5	20	Oxic	Heberer et al.,(2003b) & Pekdeger (2006)

+ Production well, ++ Monitoring well

Table 2.3 (continued)

Name	Type	Source/well	Distance (meter)	Residence time (day)	Redox conditions	References
Lake Wannsee[11]	LBF	Lake Wannsee /3335[++]	16	<30	Oxic	Heberer et al.,(2003b) & Pekdeger (2006)
Lake Wannsee[12]	LBF	Lake Wannsee /Br#4[+]	33	45	Anoxic	Heberer et al.,(2003b) & Pekdeger (2006)
Lake Wannsee[13]	LBF	Lake Wannsee /BE206[++]	1.5	15	Oxic	Grünheid and Jekel (2005)
Lake Wannsee[14]	LBF	Lake Wannsee /BE205[++]	20	15	Anoxic	Grünheid and Jekel (2005)
Lake Wannsee[15]	LBF	Lake Wannsee /BE202OP[++]		72	Oxic	Grünheid and Jekel (2005)
Lake Wannsee[16]	LBF	Lake Wannsee /BE203[++]		84	Oxic	Grünheid and Jekel (2005)
Lake Wannsee[17]	LBF	Lake Wannsee / well#3[+]	75	90	Anoxic	Heberer et al. (2008)
Lake Wannsee[18]	LBF	Lake Wannsee / BE205[++]	20	~30	Anoxic	Heberer et al. (2008)
Lake Wannsee[19]	LBF	Lake Wannsee /BE206[++]	1.5	<30	Oxic	Heberer et al. (2008)
Lake Wannsee[20]	LBF	Lake Wannsee /BE202OP[++]		60-120	Oxic	Heberer et al. (2008)
Lake Wannsee[21]	LBF	Lake Wannsee /BE203[++]		60-120	Oxic	Heberer et al. (2008)
Lake Wannsee[22]	LBF	Lake Wannsee /BE205[++]	20	~30	Anoxic	Mechlinski and Heberer (2005)
Lake Wannsee[23]	LBF	Lake Wannsee /well#3[+]	75	>120	Anoxic	Mechlinski and Heberer (2005)
Lake Wannsee[24]	LBF	Lake Wannsee /well#3[+]	75	>120	Anoxic	Heberer et al.(2003a)
Lake Wannsee[25]	LBF	Lake Wannsee /well#4[+]	100	>120	Anoxic	Heberer et al.(2003a)
Lake Wannsee[26]	LBF	Lake Wannsee /well#5[+]		>120	Anoxic	Heberer et al.(2003a)
Rhine A	RBF	Rhine/[+]	160	7-20	Oxic	Schmidt et al. (2007)
Rhine B	RBF	Rhine/[+]	70	12-60	Anoxic	Schmidt et al. (2007)
Elbe	RBF	Elbe/[+]	270	45-300	Anoxic	Schmidt et al. (2007)
Ruhr	RBF	Ruhr/[+]	125	5-15	Anaerobic	Schmidt et al. (2007)
Tucson-WR205	AR	Secondary effluent		2190		Drewes et al. (2002)
Mesa-NW2	AR	Tertiary effluent/[++]		360		Mansell and Drewes (2004a)
Mesa-NW4	AR	Tertiary effluent/[++]		540		Mansell and Drewes (2004a)
Mesa-2U	AR	Tertiary effluent/[+]		724		Mansell and Drewes (2004a)
Mesa-6U	AR	Tertiary effluent/[++]		2920		Mansell and Drewes (2004a)
Column1, 2, 3	column	Colorado River water	2.8			Snyder et al. (2007)
Column 4	column	Lake Tegel water	30	30	Oxic	Jekel and Grünheid (2005)
Column 5	column	Lake Tegel water	30	39	Anoxic	Jekel and Grünheid (2005)

+ Production well, ++ Monitoring well

2.6. Conclusions

MAR systems like BF and AR, can potentially be included in a multi-barrier treatment system for PhACs removal in drinking water treatment as part of indirect potable reuse schemes. Based on previous studies reviewed in this Chapter, the following conclusions can be drawn:

- TOC and DOC reductions for BF and AR varied from site to site, and generally, TOC and DOC removal efficiencies ranged from 30 to 88% and 33 to 88%, respectively.

- The preferential removal of non-humic substances (i.e., aliphatic organic matter or biopolymers) was observed during soil passage as a result of biodegradation.

- Ionic interactions may be a key factor in sorption mechanism for acidic pharmaceuticals such as non-steroidal anti-inflammatory drugs and lipid regulators. Thus, log D should be used to explain the fate of acidic PhACs during BF and AR.

- Antibiotics, non-steroidal anti-inflammatory drugs (NSAIDs), beta blockers and steroid hormones generally exhibited good removal efficiencies, especially for compounds having hydrophobic-neutral characteristics.

- Anticonvulsant drugs are generally difficult to remove by BF and AR.

- Pheanzone-type pharmaceuticals (NSAIDs) exhibited better removal efficiency under oxic conditions except AMDOPH which was persistent under all conditions during BF and AR.

- Some PhACs showed no significant removal under oxic conditions, including X-ray contrast agents (AOI) and sulfamethoxazole, but these compounds were removed under anoxic conditions.

- Biodegradation plays an important role in removing PhACs during soil passage.

- BF is effective for removal of redox dependent PhACs because redox conditions during BF gradually changes from oxic to anoxic during soil passage.

2.7. References

Alexander, M., 1981. Biodegradation of chemicals of environmental concern. Science 211 (4478), 132-138.

Amy, G. and Drewes, J., 2007. Soil aquifer treatment (SAT) as natural and sustainable wastewater reclamation/reuse technology: Fate of wastewater effluent organic matter (EfOM) and trace organic compounds. Environ. Monit. Assess. 129 (1-3), 19-26.

Barker, D.J. and Stuckey, D.C., 1999. A review of soluble microbial products (SMP) in wastewater treatment systems. Water Res. 33 (14), 3063-3082.

Bourg, A.C.M. and Bertin, C., 1993. Biogeochemical processes during the infiltration of river water into an alluvial aquifer. Environ. Sci. Technol. 27 (4), 661-666.

Boxall, A.B.A., Kay, P., Blackwell, P.A. and Fogg, L.A., 2004. Fate of veterinary medicines applied to soils. Springer, Berlin.

Buser, H.-R., Poiger, T. and Muller, M.D., 1999. Occurrence and environmental behavior of the chiral pharmaceutical drug ibuprofen in surface waters and in wastewater. Environ. Sci. Technol. 33 (15), 2529-2535.

Castiglioni, S., Bagnati, R., Fanelli, R., Pomati, F., Calamari, D. and Zuccato, E., 2005. Removal of pharmaceuticals in sewage treatment plants in Italy. Environ. Sci. Technol. 40 (1), 357-363.

Cha, W., Choi, H., Kim, J. and Kim, I. S., 2004. Evaluation of wastewater effluents for soil aquifer treatment in South Korea. Water Sci. Technol., 50 (2), 315-322.

Chefetz, B., Mualem, T. and Ben-Ari, J., 2008. Sorption and mobility of pharmaceutical compounds in soil irrigated with reclaimed wastewater. Chemosphere 73 (8), 1335-1343.

Chen, W., Westerhoff, P., Leenheer, J.A. and Booksh, K., 2003. Fluorescence excitation-emission matrix regional integration to quantify spectra for dissolved organic matter. Environ. Sci. Technol. 37 (24), 5701-5710.

Clara, M., Strenn, B. and Kreuzinger, N., 2004. Carbamazepine as a possible anthropogenic marker in the aquatic environment: investigations on the behaviour of carbamazepine in wastewater treatment and during groundwater infiltration. Water Res. 38 (4), 947-954.

Coble, P.G., 1996. Characterization of marine and terrestrial DOM in seawater using excitation-emission matrix spectroscopy. Mar. Chem. 51 (4), 325-346.

Cordy, G.E., Duran, N.L., Bouwer, H., Rice, R.C., Furlong, E.T., Zaugg, S.D., Meyer, M.T., Barber, L.B. and Kolpin, D.W., 2004. Do pharmaceuticals, pathogens, and other organic wast water compounds persist when waste water is used for recharge? Ground Water Monit. R. 24 (2), 58-69.

Ćosović, B., Hršak, D., Vojvodić, V. and Krznarić, D., 1996. Transformation of organic matter and bank filtration from a polluted stream. Water Res. 30 (12), 2921-2928.

Cunningham, V.L., 2004. Special characteristics of pharmaceuticals related to environmental fate. Springer, Berlin.

Cunningham, V.L., Buzby, M., Hutchinson, T., Mastrocco, F., Parke, N. and Roden, N., 2006. Effects of human pharmaceuticals on aquatic life: next steps. Environ. Sci. Technol. 40 (11), 3456-3462.

Dordio, A.V., Estevao Candeias, A.J., Pinto, A.P., Teixeira da Costa, C., Palace and Carvalho, A.J., 2009. Preliminary media screening for application in the removal of clofibric acid, carbamazepine and ibuprofen by SSF-constructed wetlands. Ecol. Eng. 35 (2), 290-302.

Drewes, J.E., Heberer, T. and Reddersen, K., 2002. Fate of pharmaceuticals during indirect potable reuse. Water Sci. Technol. 46 (3), 73-80.

Eckert, P. and Irmscher R., 2006. Practical Paper Over 130 years of experience with riverbank Filtration in Dusseldorf, Germany. J. Water Supply Res. T. 55 (4), 283-291.

Gebhardt, W. and Schröer, H.F., 2007. Liquid chromatography-(tandem) mass spectrometry for the follow-up of the elimination of persistent pharmaceuticals during wastewater treatment applying biological wastewater treatment and advanced oxidation. J. Chromatogr., A 1160 (1-2), 34-43.

Grünheid, S., Amy, G. and Jekel, M., 2005. Removal of bulk dissolved organic carbon (DOC) and trace organic compounds by bank filtration and artificial recharge. Water Res. 39 (14), 3219.

Grünheid, S. and Jekel, M., 2005. Fate of bulk organics during bank filtration of wastewater-impacted surface water. In: Proceedings of the 5th international symposium on management of aquifer recharge, Berlin, 10-16 June 2005.

Grützmacher, G., Hülshoff, I., Wiese, B., Golvan, Y., Sprenger, C., Lorenzen, G. and Pekdeger, A., 2009. Function and relevance of aquifer recharge techniques to enable sustainable water resources management in developing or newly-industrialized countries. IWA publishing.

Gupta, V., Johnson, W.P., Shafieian, P., Ryu, H., Alum, A., Abbaszadegan, M., Hubbs, S.A. and Rauch-Williams, T., 2009. Riverbank filtration: comparison of pilot scale transport with theory. Environ. Sci. Technol. 43 (8), 2992-2992.

Heberer, T., 2002. Occurrence, fate, and removal of pharmaceutical residues in the aquatic environment: a review of recent research data. Toxicol. Lett. 131 (1-2), 5-17.

Heberer, T. and Adam, M., 2004. Transport and Attenuation of Pharmaceutical Residues During Artificial Groundwater Replenishment. Environ. Chem. 1 (1), 22-25.

Heberer, T., Fanck, B., Mechlinski, A., Zühlke, S., Adam, M., Voigt, M., Wicke, D. and Dünnbier, U., 2003a Occurrence and Fate of Drug Residues and Related Polar Contaminants during Bank Filtration. Berlin Centre for Water Competence, Berlin.

Heberer, T., Mechlinski, A. and Fanck, B., 2003b. NASRI - Occurrence and Fate of Pharmaceuticals during Bank Filtration. Conference Wasser Berlin 2003, Berlin Centre for Water Competence, Berlin.

Heberer, T., Massmann, G., Fanck, B., Taute, T. and Dünbier, U., 2008. Behaviour and redox sensitivity of antimicrobial residues during bank filtration. Chemosphere 73 (4), 451-460.

Heberer, T., Mechlinski, A., Fanck, B., Knappe, A., Massmann, G., Pekdeger, A. and Fritz, B., 2004. Field Studies on the Fate and Transport of Pharmaceutical Residues in Bank Filtration. Ground Water Monit. R. 24 (2), 70-77.

Heberer, T., Reddersen, K., and Mechlinski, A., 2002. From municipal sewage to drinking water: fate and removal of pharmaceutical residues in the aquatic environment in urban areas. Water Sci. Technol. 46 (3), 81-88.

Henderson, R.K., Baker, A., Murphy, K.R., Hambly, A., Stuetz, R.M. and Khan, S.J., 2009. Fluorescence as a potential monitoring tool for recycled water systems: A review. Water Res. 43 (3), 863-881.

Hiemstra, P., Kolpa, R.J., Eekhout, J.M.J.M.v., Kessel, T.A.L.v., Adamse, E.D. and Paassen, J.A.M.v., 2003. Natural recharge of groundwater: bank infiltration in the Netherlands. J. Water Supply Res. T. 52 (1), 37-47.

Hiscock, K.M. and Grischek, T., 2002. Attenuation of groundwater pollution by bank filtration. J. Hydrol. 266 (3-4), 139-144.

Howard, P.H., 2000. Biodegradation. Handbook of property estimation methods for chemicals and health sciences. CRC Press LLC, Boca Raton.

Huber, S. and Frimmel, F.H., 1992. A liquid chromatographic system with multi-detection for the direct analysis of hydrophilic organic compounds in natural waters. Fresenius J. Anal. Chem. 342 (1-2), 198-200.

Irmscher, R. and Teermann, I., 2002. Riverbank filtration for drinking water supply - a proven method, perfect to face today's challenge. Water Sci. Technol. 2 (5-6), 1-8.

Jarusutthirak, C. and Amy, G., 2006. Role of soluble microbial products (SMP) in membrane fouling and flux decline. Environ. Sci. Technol. 40 (3), 969-974.

Jekel, M. and Grünheid, S., 2003. NASRI-Removal of organic substances. In: Proceedings of the conference Wasser Berlin, 7-11 April 2003.

Jekel, M. and Grünheid, S., 2005. Bank filtration and groundwater recharge for treatment of polluted surface waters. Water Sci. Technol. 5 (5), 57-66.

Jjemba, P.K., 2006. Excretion and ecotoxicity of pharmaceutical and personal care products in the environment. Ecotox. Environ. Safe. 63 (1), 113-130.

Kagle, J., Porter, A.W., Murdoch, R.W., Rivera-Cancel, G., Hay, A.G., 2009. Biodegradation of pharmaceuticals and personal care products. Adv. Appl. Microbiol. 67, 65-108.

Kasprzyk-Hordern, B., Dinsdale, R.M., and Guwy, A.J., 2009. The removal of pharmaceuticals, personal care products, endocrine disruptors and illicit drugs during wastewater treatment and its impact on the quality of receiving waters. Water Res. 43 (2), 363-380.

Kedziorek, M.A.M., Geoffriau, S. and Bourg, A.C.M., 2008. Organic matter and modeling redox reactions during river bank filtration in an alluvial aquifer of the Lot River, France. Environ. Sci. Technol. 42 (8), 2793-2798.

Kim, S.D., Cho, J., Kim, I.S., Vanderford, B.J. and Snyder, S.A., 2007. Occurrence and removal of pharmaceuticals and endocrine disruptors in South Korean surface, drinking, and waste waters. Water Res. 41 (5), 1013-1021.

Klavarioti, M., Mantzavinos, D., and Kassinos, D., 2009. Removal of residual pharmaceuticals from aqueous systems by advanced oxidation processes. Environ. Int. 35 (2), 402-417.

Kolehmainen, R.E., Langwaldt, J.g.H. and Puhakka, J.A., 2007. Natural organic matter (NOM) removal and structural changes in the bacterial community during artificial groundwater recharge with humic lake water. Water Res. 41 (12), 2715-2725.

Kümmerer, K., 2009. The presence of pharmaceuticals in the environment due to human use - present knowledge and future challenges. J. Environ. Manage. 90 (8), 2354-2366.

Lee, J.-H., Hamm, S.-Y., Cheong, J.-Y., Kim, H.-S., Ko, E.-J., Lee, K.-S. and Lee, S.-I., 2009. Characterizing riverbank-filtered water and river water qualities at a site in the lower Nakdong River basin, Republic of Korea. J. Hydrol. 376 (1-2), 209-220.

Leenheer, J.A. and Croue, J.-P., 2003. Characterizing aquatic dissolved organic matter. Environ. Sci. Technol. 37 (1), 18A-26A.

Lin, A.Y.-C., Plumlee, M.H., and Reinhard, M., 2006. Natural attenuation of pharmaceuticals and alkylphenol polyethoxylate metabolites during river transport: photochemical and biological transformation. Environ. Toxicol. Chem. 25 (6), 1458-1464.

Madden, J.C., Enoch, S.J., Hewitt, M. and Cronin, M.T.D., 2009. Pharmaceuticals in the environment: Good practice in predicting acute ecotoxicological effects. Toxicol. Lett. 185 (2), 85-101.

Maeng, S.K., Sharma, S.K., Amy, G. and Magic-Knezev, A., 2008. Fate of effluent organic matter (EfOM) and natural organic matter (NOM) through riverbank filtration. Water Sci. Technol. 57 (12), 1999–2007.

Mansell, J. and Drewes, J.E., 2004a. Fate of steroidal hormones during soil-aquifer treatment. Ground Water Monit. R. 24 (2), 94-101.

Mansell, J., Drewes, J.E. and Rauch, T., 2004b. Removal mechanism of endocrine disrupting compounds (steroids) soil aquifer treatment. Water Sci. Technol. 50 (2), 229-237.

Massmann, G., Dunnbier, U., Heberer, T. and Taute, T., 2008. Behaviour and redox sensitivity of pharmaceutical residues during bank filtration - Investigation of residues of phenazone-type analgesics. Chemosphere 71 (8), 1476-1485.

Massmann, G., Greskowiak, J., Dünnbier, U. and Zuehlke, S., 2006. The impact of variable temperatures on the redox conditions and the behavior of pharmaceutical residues during artificial recharge. J. Hydrol. 328 (1-2), 141-156.

Matamoros, V.t., Caselles-Osorio, A., Garc, J. and Bayona, J.M., 2008. Behaviour of pharmaceutical products and biodegradation intermediates in horizontal subsurface flow constructed wetland. A microcosm experiment. Sci. Total Environ. 394 (1), 171-176.

Mechlinski, A. and Heberer, T., 2005. Fate and transport of pharmaceutical residues during bank filtration. In: Proceedings of 5th international symposium on management of aquifer recharge, Berlin, 10-16 June 2005.

Metcalfe, C., Miao, X.-S., Hua, W., Letcher, R., Servos, M., 2004. Pharmaceuticals in the Canadian environment. Springer, Berlin.

Mompelat, S., LeBot, B. and Thomas, O., 2009. Occurrence and fate of pharmaceutical products and by-products, from resource to drinking water. Environ. Int. 35 (5), 803-814.

Nederlof, M.M., Kruithof, J.C., Taylor, J.S., van der Kooij, D. and Schippers, J.C., 2000. Comparison of NF/RO membrane performance in integrated membrane systems. Desalination 131 (1-3), 257-269.

Partinoudi, V. and Collins M.R., 2007. Assessing RBF reduction/removal mechanisms for microbial and organic DBP precursors. J. AWWA 99, 61-71.

Pekdeger, A., 2006. Hydrogeological-hydrogeochemical processes during bank filtration and groundwater recharge using a multi-tracer approach. NASRI Project, Berlin.

Philibert, M., Bush, S., and Rosario-Ortiz, F.L. and Suffet, I.H., 2008. Advances in the characterization of the polarity of DOM under ambient water quality conditions using the polarity rapid assessment method. Water Sci. Technol. 8 (6), 725-733.

Quanrud, D.M., Hafer, J., Karpiscak, M.M., Zhang, J., Lansey, K.E. and Arnold, R.G., 2003. Fate of organics during soil-aquifer treatment: sustainability of removals in the field. Water Res. 37 (14), 3401-3411.

Radjenovic, J., Petrovic, M., Ventura, F. and Barcel, D., 2008. Rejection of pharmaceuticals in nanofiltration and reverse osmosis membrane drinking water treatment. Water Res. 42 (14), 3601-3610.

Rauch, T. and Drewes, J.E., 2004. Assessing the removal potential of soil-aquifer treatment systems for bulk organic matter. Water Sci. Technol. 50 (2), 245-253.

Ray, C., 2008. Worldwide potential of riverbank filtration. Clean Technol. Envir. 10 (3), 223-225.

Ray, C., Grischek, T., Schubert, J., Wang, J. and Speth, T., 2002a. A perspective of riverbank filtration. J. AWWA 94 (3), 149-160.

Ray, C., Schubert, J., Linsky, R.B. and Melin, G., 2002b. Introduction. Riverbank filtration: Improving source-water quality. In: Ray, C., Melin, G., Linsky, R.B. (Ed.). Kluwer Academic Publishers, Dordrecht.

Ray, C., Soong, T.W., Lian, Y.Q. and Roadcap, G.S., 2002c. Effect of flood-induced chemical load on filtrate quality at bank filtration sites. J. Hydrol. 266 (3-4), 235-258.

Rosario-Ortiz, F.L., Gerringer, F.W. and Suffet, I.H., 2009. Application of a novel polarity method for the characterization of natural organic matter during water treatment. J. Water Supply Res. T. 58 (3), 159-169.

Rosario-Ortiz, F.L., Kozawa, K., Al-Samarrai, H.N., Gerringer, F.W., Gabelich, C.J. and Suffet, I.H., 2004. Characterization of the changes in polarity of natural organic matter using solid-phase extraction: introducing the NOM polarity rapid assessment method (NOM-PRAM). Water Sci. Technol. 40 (4), 11-18.

Rosario-Ortiz, F.L., Snyder, S. and Suffet, I.H., 2007a. Characterization of the polarity of natural organic matter under ambient conditions by the polarity rapid assessment method (PRAM). Environ. Sci. Technol. 41 (14), 4895-4900.

Rosario-Ortiz, F.L., Snyder, S.A. and Suffet, I.H., 2007b. Characterization of dissolved organic matter in drinking water sources impacted by multiple tributaries. Water Res. 41 (18), 4115-4128.

Schittko, S., Putschew, A. and Jekel, M., 2004. Bank filtration: a suitable process for the removal of iodinated X-ray contrast media. Water Sci. Technol. 50 (5), 261-268.

Schmidt, C.K., Lange, F.T. and Brauch, H.J., 2007. Characteristics and evaluation of natural attenuation processes for organic micropollutant removal during riverbank filtration. In: Proceedings of the Regional IWA conference on groundwater management in the Danube River Basin and other large River Basins, Belgrade, 7-9 June 2007.

Schmidt, C., Lange, F., Brauch, H. and Kuhn, W., 2003. Experiences with riverbank filtration and infiltration in Germany. International symposium on artificial recharge of groundwater. K-WATER, Daejon, Korea, pp. 117–131.

Schoenheinz, D., Bornick, H. and Worch, E., 2005. Temperature effects on organics removal during river bank filtration. In: Proceedings of the 5th international symposium on management of aquifer recharge, Berlin, 10-16 June 2005.

Schubert, J., 2002. Water-quality improvements with riverbank filtration at Dusseldorf waterworks in Germany. In: Chittaranjan, R., Melin, G., Linsky, R.B. (Eds.). Riverbank filtration: Improving source-water quality. Kluwer Academic Publishers, Dordrecht.

Shamrukh, M. and Abdel-Wahab, A., 2008. Riverbank filtration for sustainable water supply: application to a large-scale facility on the Nile River. Clean Technol. Envir. 10 (4), 351-358.

Snyder, S.A., Leising, J., Westerhoff, P., Yoon, Y., Mash, H. and Vanderford, B., 2004. Biological and Physical Attenuation of Endocrine Disruptors and Pharmaceuticals: Implications for Water Reuse. Ground Water Monit. R. 24 (2), 108-118.

Snyder, S.A., Wert, E.C., Lei, H., Westerhoff, P. and Yoon, Y., 2007. Removal of EDCs and pharmaceuticals in drinking and reuse treatment processes. AwwaRF, Denver.

Speth, T.F., Merkel, T. and Gusses, A.M., 2002. Riverbank filtration as a pretreatment for nanofiltration membranes. In: Ray, C., Melin, G., Linsky, R.B. (Eds.). Riverbank filtration: Improving source-water quality. Kluwer Academic Publishers, Dordrecht.

Stamatelatou, K., Frouda, C., Fountoulakis, M.S., Drillia, P., Kornaros, M. and Lyberatos, G., 2003. Pharmaceuticals and health care products in wastewater effluents: the example of carbamazepine. Water Sci. Technol: Water Supply 3 (4), 131-137.

Ternes, T.A., 1998. Occurence of drugs in German sewage treatment plants and rivers. Water Res. 32 (11), 3245-3260.

Ternes, T.A., Bonerz, M., Herrmann, N., Teiser, B. and Andersen, H.R., 2007. Irrigation of treated wastewater in Braunschweig, Germany: An option to remove pharmaceuticals and musk fragrances. Chemosphere 66 (5), 894-904.

Ternes, T.A., Meisenheimer, M., McDowell, D., Sacher, F., Brauch, H.J., Haist-Gulde, B., Preuss, G., Wilme, U. and Zulei-Seibert, N., 2002. Removal of pharmaceuticals during drinking water treatment. Environ. Sci. Technol. 36 (17), 3855-3863.

Tixier, C., Singer, H.P., Oellers, S. and Muller, S.R., 2003. Occurrence and fate of carbamazepine, clofibric acid, diclofenac, ibuprofen, ketoprofen, and naproxen in surface waters. Environ. Sci. Technol. 37 (16), 1061-1068.

Tufenkji, N., Ryan, J.N. and Elimelech, M., 2002. The promise of bank filtration. Environ. Sci. Technol. 36 (21), 422A-428A.

US EPA, 2009. Estimation Programs Interface Suite™ for Microsoft® Windows, v 4.00. United States Environmental Protection Agency, Washington, DC, USA.

Verstraeten, I. M., Heberer, T. and Scheytt, T. 2002. Occurrence, characteristics, andtransport and fate of pesticides, pharmaceutical active compounds, and industrial and personal care products at bank-filtration sites. In: Riverbank Filtration: Improving Source-Water Quality, Kluwer Academic Publishers, Dordrecht, 175-227.

Wang, J., Hubbs, S.A. and Song, R., 2002. Evaluation of riverbank filtration as a drinking water treatment process. AWWA Research Foundation and AWWA.

Weiss, W.J., Bouwer, E.J., Ball, W.P., O'Melia, C.R., Aboytes., R. and Speth, T.F., 2004. Riverbank filtration: Effect of ground passage on NOM character. J. Water Supply Res. T. 53 (2), 61-83.

Weiss, W.J., Bouwer, E.J., Ball, W.P., O'Melia, C.R., Arora, H. and Speth, T.F., 2002. Reduction in Disinfection Byproduct Precursors and Pathogens During Riverbank Filtration at Three Midwestern United States Drinking-Water Utilities. In: Ray, C., Melin, G., Linsky, R.B. (Eds.). Riverbank filtration-improving source-water quality. Kluwer Academic Publishers, Dordrecht.

Wick, A., Fink, G., Joss, A., Siegrist, H., Ternes and T.A., 2009. Fate of beta blockers and psycho-active drugs in conventional wastewater treatment. Water Res. 43 (4), 1060-1074.

Winkler, M., Lawrence, J.R. and Neu, T.R., 2001. Selective degradation of ibuprofen and clofibric acid in two model river biofilm systems. Water Res. 35 (13), 3197-3205.

Wu, Y., Hui, L., Wang, H., Li, Y. and Zeng, R., 2007. Effectiveness of riverbank filtration for removal of nitrogen from heavily polluted rivers: a case study of Kuihe River, Xuzhou, Jiangsu, China Environ. Geol. 52 (1), 19-25.

Xue, S., Zhao, Q.L., Wei, L.L. and Ren, N.Q., 2009. Behavior and characteristics of dissolved organic matter during column studies of soil aquifer treatment, Water Res., 43 (2), 499-507,

Yangali-Quintanilla, V., Sadmani, A., McConville, M., Kennedy, M. and Amy, G., 2009. Rejection of pharmaceutically active compounds and endocrine disrupting compounds by clean and fouled nanofiltration membranes. Water Res. 43 (9), 2349-2362.

Ying, G.-G., Kookana, R.S. and Dillon, P., 2003. Sorption and degradation of selected five endocrine disrupting chemicals in aquifer material. Water Res. 37 (15), 3785-3791.

Yoon, Y., Westerhoff, P., Snyder, S.A. and Wert, E.C., 2006. Nanofiltration and ultrafiltration of endocrine disrupting compounds, pharmaceuticals and personal care products. J. Membrane Sci. 270 (1-2), 88-100.

Zhang, Y., Geissen, S.-U. and Gal, C., 2008. Carbamazepine and diclofenac: Removal in wastewater treatment plants and occurrence in water bodies. Chemosphere 73 (8), 1151-1161.

Zhou, J.L., Zhang, Z.L., Banks, E., Grover, D. and Jiang, J.Q., 2009. Pharmaceutical residues in wastewater treatment works effluents and their impact on receiving river water. Journal of Hazardous Materials 166 (2-3), 655-661.

Zuehlke,S., Duennbier, U., Heberer, T. and Fritz, B., 2004. Analysis of endocrine disrupting steroids: Investigation of their Release into the environment and their behavior during bank filtration." Ground Water Monit. R. 24(2), 78-85.

Zuehlke, S., Duennbier, U. and Heberer, T., 2007. Investigation of the behavior and metabolism of pharmaceutical residues during purification of contaminated ground water used for drinking water supply. Chemosphere 69 (11), 1673-1680.

Chapter 3
FATE OF EFFLUENT ORGANIC MATTER DURING BANK FILTRATION

Parts of this chapter were based on:

Maeng, S.K., Sharma, S.K., Amy, G.L. and Magic-Knezev, A., 2008. Fate of effluent organic matter (EfOM) and natural organic matter (NOM) through riverbank filtration. Water Science & Technology. 57(12), 1999–2007.

Baghoth, S.A., Maeng, S.K., Salinas Rodríguez, S.G., Ronteltap, M., Sharma S.K., Kennedy M. and Amy, G.L., 2008. An urban water cycle perspective of natural organic matter (NOM): NOM in drinking water, wastewater effluent, storm water, and seawater, Water Science & Technology: Water Supply 6(8), 701-707.

Sharma S.K., Baghoth, S.A., Maeng, S.K., Salinas Rodríguez, S.G., Amy, G.L, 2011. Chapter 3. Natural Organic Matter: Characterization Profiling as a Basis for Treatment Process Selection and Performance Monitoring. In "Handbook on Particle Separation Processes", A. van Nieuwenhuijzen and J. van der Graaf (eds.), IWA Publications (In Press).

Summary

Understanding the fate of effluent organic matter (EfOM) and natural organic matter (NOM) through bank filtration (BF) is essential to assess the impact of wastewater effluent on the post treatment requirements of bank filtrates. Column studies were conducted to characterize bulk organic matter which consists of EfOM and NOM during BF using a suite of innovative analytical tools and to determine the removal of selected pharmaceutically active compounds (PhACs). Results showed the preferential removal of non-humic substances (i.e., biopolymers) from wastewater effluent-impacted surface water. The bulk organic matter characteristics of wastewater effluent-impacted surface water and surface water were similar after 5 m soil passage. Humic-like organic matter in surface water and wastewater effluent-impacted surface water persisted through the soil passage. More than 50% of total dissolved organic carbon (DOC) removal with significant reduction of dissolved oxygen (DO) was observed in the top 50 cm of the soil columns. This was due to biodegradation by soil biomass which was determined by measuring adenosine triphosphate (ATP) concentrations and heterotrophic plate counts. Good correlation of DOC removal with DO and biomass development was observed in the soil columns. DOC removal was lower under anoxic conditions compared to oxic conditions. Most of the selected PhACs exhibited removal efficiencies greater than 90% in both wastewater effluent-impacted surface water and surface water. However, removal efficiencies of bezafibrate, diclofenac, and gemfibrozil were relatively low in wastewater effluent-impacted surface water. This result indicates that EfOM characteristics or microbial diversity affect biotransformation of some PhACs. Further study is needed to define microorganisms responsible for the biotransformation of PhACs. Carbamazepine and clofibric acid showed a persistent behavior and were not influenced by EfOM removal. The removal efficiencies of selected PhACs in this study did not vary under different redox conditions.

3.1. Introduction

Bank filtration (BF) is a natural treatment process for drinking water. BF systems induce surface water to flow in response to a hydraulic gradient through intake facilities such as vertical, horizontal or angle well types by lowering the water level. It is a relatively robust and multi-objective barrier that has sufficient buffer capacity to chemical shock loads or temperature changes. In North America, riverbank filtration (RBF) is given 1.0 log removal credit for *Cryptosporidium* by U.S. Environmental Protection Agency if the RBF system is designed and constructed according to USEPA guidance (USEPA, 2003). This has triggered some water utilities in North America to investigate the feasibility of a RBF system for part of their treatment steps to improve their raw water quality. In contrast, many cities along the River Rhine have been successfully supplying drinking water treated through BF for many years. BF has been practiced in Europe for more than 100 years in water treatment systems (Eckert and Irmscher, 2006). BF is becoming a part of a multi barrier system in a drinking water treatment scheme to remove emerging wastewater-derived organic micropollutants (OMPs) such as pharmaceutically active compounds (PhACs) and endocrine disrupting compounds (EDCs). BF is also an attractive water treatment process for developing countries because it is a relatively cost-effective, robust and sustainable technology. Most water utilities in developing countries have a conventional water treatment process or less and their surface waters are often influenced by wastewater. Many developing countries discharge their sewage into the aquatic environment without any treatment or just after primary treatment. The influence of wastewater on drinking water resources is not only a problem for developing countries but also for developed countries because they have to cope with effluent organic matter (EfOM) in wastewater effluent which is discharged into the river.

EfOM has not been extensively studied compared to natural organic matter (NOM). EfOM is composed of different types of organics: refractory compounds, residual degradable substrate, intermediates, complex organic compounds, and soluble microbial products (SMPs) (Barker and Stuckey, 1999). The characteristics of EfOM that remains after secondary treatment is quite different from that of untreated wastewater (Levine et al., 1985). EfOM does not pose a direct health threat to humans in terms of drinking water quality, but it has a more biodegradable organic fraction compared to that of NOM. SMPs, produced by microorganisms as part of the metabolism in degrading EfOM, is a factor in membrane fouling of reverse osmosis (RO), nano filtration (NF), and tight ultra filtration (UF) membranes (Jarusutthirak and Amy, 2006). SMPs such as polysaccharides and proteins in EfOM can be also used as a substrate for the regrowth of microorganisms in a distribution system, however the kinetics of degradation may be considerably slower than simple substrates (Barker and Stuckey, 1999). EfOM also consists of humic substances which are derived from the drinking water source and serve as a precursor to disinfection by-product (DBPs) while SMPs (proteins) in EfOM represent a precursor to nitrogenous DBPs (N-DBPs) (Amy and Drews, 2007). Bulk organic matter in wastewater effluent-impacted surface water consists of both anthropogenic (EfOM) and allochthonous (NOM) characteristics.

Redox conditions during BF gradually change from oxic to anoxic/anaerobic, and the transition of redox conditions is dependent on water quality, residence times and travel distances. Grünheid et al. (2005) elucidated that the fate of bulk organic matter is different under different redox conditions. They found that in contrast to oxic conditions, specific UV absorbance (SUVA) values decreased under anoxic conditions which imply that the degradation of aromatic organic matter was relatively higher. Redox conditions not only affect the fate of bulk organic matter but also the behavior of wastewater derived OMPs during soil passage. For example, some PhACs (e.g., phenazone and sulfamethoxazole) are redox dependent compounds; thus, their removals vary with redox conditions (Massmann et al., 2006; Schmidt et al., 2007).

There has been a growing concern over the increased detection of OMPs including PhACs, EDCs, and personal care products (PCPs), in drinking water sources, especially in the downstream of the river when secondary effluent (SE) is discharged from wastewater treatment plants. The occurrence of OMPs in drinking water sources has resulted in increased research in developing innovative water treatment technologies to provide reliable supply of safe drinking water to customers (Kim et al., 2007; Madden et al., 2009; Mechlinski and Heberer, 2005; Mompelat et al., 2009). Installing an additional treatment process for the removal of OMPs is relatively costly for water utilities and may result in increasing the price of drinking water. Managed aquifer recharge (MAR) processes such as BF, lake bank filtration (LBF) and artificial recharge (AR) are robust and cost-effective treatments for OMP removals. Previous studies have shown that MAR systems are effective for removal of some OMPs (Grünheid and Jekel, 2005; Heberer et al., 2004; Massmann et al., 2008; Mechlinski and Heberer, 2005).

Several studies in the past attempted to examine the fate of EfOM during MAR. However, there has been no research on: 1) comparison on the fate of bulk organic matter characteristics between wastewater effluent-impacted surface water and surface water during soil passage: 2) the impact of EfOM on the removal of PhACs during soil passage. The objective of this study was to investigate the fate of bulk organic matter characteristics during soil passage under different redox conditions in wastewater effluent-impacted surface water. Moreover, this study investigated the effects of EfOM on the removal of different classes of PhACs. Adenosine triphosphate (ATP) at different depths of the soil columns provided insight into the role of microbial activity on the fate of bulk organic matter and selected PhACs during soil passage.

3.2. Materials and Methods

3.2.1. Chemicals

13 PhACs were used to prepare stock solutions, out of which working solutions were made and spiked into soil column setups. All PhACs under investigation were of analytical grade (> 90%) and purchased from Sigma–Aldrich, Germany (gemfibrozil, diclofenac, bezafibrate, ibuprofen, fenoprofen, naproxen, ketoprofen, clofibric acid, carbamazepine, phenacetine, paracetamol, pentoxifylline and caffeine). The physicochemical properties of selected compounds are shown in Table 3.1.

Table 3.1 Physicochemical properties of selected pharmaceutically active compounds

Name	MW (g/mol)	pK_a	log K_{ow}[1]	log D^2 (pH=8)	Charge @ pH=8[3]
Gemfibrozil	250.3	4.7	4.77	2.22	Hydrophobic-Ionic
Diclofenac	296.2	4.2	4.51	1.59	Hydrophilic-Ionic
Bezafibrate	361.8	3.6	4.25	0.69	Hydrophilic-Ionic
Ibuprofen	206.3	4.9	3.97	1.44	Hydrophilic-Ionic
Fenoprofen	242.3	4.5	3.9	1.11	Hydrophilic-Ionic
Naproxen	230.3	4.2	3.18	0.05	Hydrophilic-Ionic
Ketoprofen	254.3	4.5	3.12	0.41	Hydrophilic-Ionic
Clofibric acid	214.6	3.2	2.88	-1.08	Hydrophilic-Ionic
Carbamazepine	236.3	N.A.[4]	2.45	N.A.[4]	Hydrophilic-Neutral
Phenacetine	179.2	N.A.[4]	1.67	N.A.[4]	Hydrophilic-Neutral
Paracetamol	151.2	N.A.[4]	0.27	N.A.[4]	Hydrophilic-Neutral
Pentoxifylline	278.3	N.A.[4]	0.29	N.A.[4]	Hydrophilic-Neutral
Caffeine	194.2	N.A.[4]	-0.07	N.A.[4]	Hydrophilic-Neutral

[1] KOWWIN v.1.67 (US EPA, 2009)
[2] ADME/Tox WEB software (http://www.pharma-algorithms.com/webboxes/)
[3] For acidic pharmaceuticals: hydrophobic: log D > 1, hydrophilic: log D < 1 at pH 8; for neutral pharmaceuticals: hydrophobic: log K_{ow} > 2, hydrophilic: K_{ow} < 2
[4] Not applicable

3.2.2. Soil column studies

Laboratory-scale column studies, simulating BF, were conducted using the experimental setup shown in Figure 3.1. Four laboratory-scale column set-ups were constructed from a PVC pipe with internal diameter of 100 mm. The bottom of each column was packed with filter media support of 15 cm thick graded gravel and then filled with clean silica sand sized between 0.8 and 1.25 mm. Each set consisted of two columns, with each 2.5 m in height, connected in series to simulate a 5 m depth of a one dimensional aquifer. Each soil column consisted of 14 sampling ports (SP) located along the columns, and a number of SP was higher in the first column than in the second column because of the biological layer formed on the top surface of a soil column (*Schmutzdecke*) which plays an important role in the transformation of bulk organic matter. The first five sampling points were placed closely to each other (SP1-SP2 = 5 cm, SP2-SP3 = 10 cm, SP3-SP4 = 10 cm, SP4-SP5 = 20 cm) and remaining sampling points were located at 50 cm intervals. The soil columns were operated under a down-flow mode, and the flow rate (hydraulic loading rate, 1.4 m/day) was controlled by the valves located at the outlet of the second columns.

All of the columns were acclimated for least 40 days using SE to stabilize soil biomass associated with sand. Stabilization of columns was ascertained with respect to constant DOC removal. Firstly, two sets of columns were used to assess effects of EfOM on the characteristics of bulk organic matter in canal water (Delft, The Netherlands) (SC1 and SC2). Secondly, another two sets of columns were used to determine effects of EfOM on the characteristics of bulk organic matter in the river (the River Meuse, Netherlands) (SC3 and SC4) (Table 3.2). Thus, surface waters, Delft canal water (DCW) and the River Meuse (MR) water, were amended with SE from WWTP (Hoek van Holland, The Netherlands) in a 1:1 ratio to simulate wastewater effluent-impacted surface water (50% of SE) for SC1 and SC4, respectively. The HLR of column setups was 1.4 m/day. All influents were filtered through a microsieve (38 μm) prior to infiltration to prevent physical clogging on the top layers of soil column.

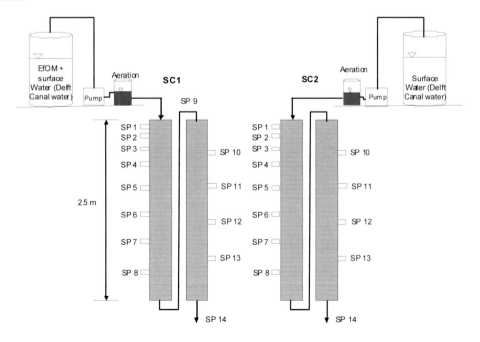

Figure 3.1 Schematic diagram of the soil column experimental setup (SC1 and SC2)

Table 3.2 Column experimental set-ups

	Influent	PhACs[4]	HLR[5] (m/d)
SC1	DCW[1]+SE[2] (1:1)	N.A.[4]	1.4
SC2	DCW	N.A.[4]	1.4
SC3	MR[3]	spiked	1.4
SC4	MR+SE (1:1)	spiked	1.4

[1]DCW: Delft canal water, [2]SE: secondary effluent, [3]MR: The River Meuse, [4] N.A.: Not Applied, [5]HLR: hydraulic loading rate

3.2.3. Analytics

All samples were stored at 4°C after 0.45 μm filtration (Whatman, Dassel, Germany) to prevent biodegradation of organic matter and were characterized within 3 days after sample collection. The concentration of bulk organic matter was determined as DOC (dissolved organic carbon) by a total organic carbon analyzer (Shimadzu TOC-V$_{CPN}$). The characteristics of bulk organic matter were elucidated by various analytical methods including fluorescence excitation-emission matrix (F-EEM), liquid chromatography with an on-line organic carbon detection and an organic nitrogen detection (LC-OCD/OND) (DOC-LABOR Dr. Huber, Karlsruhe, Germany) and specific ultraviolet absorbance (SUVA). For F-EEM analysis, all samples were adjusted to pH 2 by diluting samples to 1 mg/L of DOC with 0.01 N KCl due to the fluorophore interferences by metals, and measured by a FluoroMax-3 spectrofluorometer (HORIBA Jobin Yvon, Edison, NJ, USA). Table 3.3 and Figure 3.2 show the characteristics of organic matter expressed as regions determined by distinct wavelengths of excitation and emission (Leenheer and Croue, 2003). LC-OCD/OND uses a liquid chromatography method describing the molecular weight (MW) distribution and classification of organic matter according to biopolymers, humics substances, building blocks, neutrals and low MW acids. Specific UV absorbance (SUVA) is the ratio between DOC and UVA at 254 nm and shows the aromaticity of humic content of the bulk organic matter.

Table 3.3 Characteristics of organic matter using 3 key fluorescence peaks (primary humic-like peak (P1), secondary humic-like peak (P2) and protein-like peak (P3)) in F-EEM

	Excitation (nm)	Emission (nm)	Description	References
P1	250-260	380-480	Humic-like substances	(Leenheer and Croue 2003)
	237-260	400-500	(Primary)	(Coble 1996)
P2	330-350	420-480	Humic-like substances	(Leenheer and Croue 2003)
	300-370	400-500	(Secondary)	(Coble 1996)
P3	270-280	320-350	Tryptophan-like,	(Leenheer and Croue 2003)
	275	340	Protein-like	(Coble 1996)
	280	350	substances	(Henderson et al. 2009)

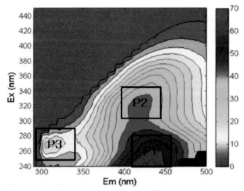

Figure 3.2 Typical F-EEM spectra from secondary effluent

For sample preparation for selected PhACs, autotrace SPE workstations from Caliper Life Sciences GmbH (Rüsselsheim, Germany) were used for solid phase extraction. GC-MS analysis was used with a GCQ from Thermo Scientific (Dreieich, Germany) equipped with a split/splitless injector and an ion-trap mass spectrometer. HPLC-ESI-MS-MS measurements were performed on a HPLC system 1100, Series II from Agilent Technologies (Waldbronn, Germany) equipped with an API 2000 triple quadrupole mass spectrometer from PE Sciex (Langen, Germany) using electrospray ionisation (ESI) under atmospheric pressure. Discussion of the details of the method is given elsewhere (Sacher et al., 2008).

3.2.4. Biomass measurement

Rauch-Williams and Drewes (2005) used soil biomass as an indicator for biodegradation of EfOM during soil infiltration. They used three methods (dehydrogenase activity (DHA), phospholipid extraction (PLE), and substrate induced respiration (SIR)) to determine how soil biomass is related to organic carbon removal. In this study, ATP was measured to determine biomass concentration (activity) in soil columns. Soil ATP is closely correlated to biomass concentration. Therefore, ATP can be used as an indicator of soil microbial biomass (Oades and Jenkinson, 1979). The ATP analysis is simple and accurate, commonly used in aquatic microbiology and is a suitable parameter for the quantification of the active biomass (Velten et al., 2007). Wet sand samples of 2 to 4 g, collected from different depths, were suspended in the autoclaved tap water (50 mL). High energy sonication at a power of 40 W was applied to detach the biomass (Branson W-250D Sonifier, microtip D = 5 mm). The biomass concentration was determined as the concentration of ATP in the suspension obtained by the sonication. A single 2-minute sonication treatment was adequate to obtain more than 90% of the attached biomass represented as ATP (data not shown). A detailed description of methods and materials used for ATP extraction procedure is explained in Magic-Knezev and van der Kooij (2004). Heterotrophic plate counts (HPC) were carried out as another biomass parameter to determine the correlation between ATP and HPC in bioactive sands. A total of 0.1 mL of microbial suspensions obtained by sonication were spread in triplicate over a surface of R_2A agar (Carl Roth, Karlsruhe, Germany) plates which were incubated for 5 days at 25 ºC.

3.3. Results and discussion

Two different types of wastewater effluent-impacted surface waters were prepared by mixing MR with SE (1:1) and DCW with SE (1:1) and were used to investigate effects of EfOM on the fate of bulk organic matter during soil passage. Firstly, DCW containing relatively high amount of humic substances, was used to simulate wastewater effluent-impacted surface water (SC1 and SC2). Two different HLRs (1.4 and 2.8 m/day) were also tested to investigate the difference in the removal of DOC. Secondly, MR, which is used as a drinking water source, was used to assess the impact of EfOM on the fate of bulk organic matter and selected PhACs during soil passage (SC3 and SC4).

3.3.1 Bulk organic matter characteristics-Canal water (SC1 and SC2)

SUVA, DOC and DO

Initially, both columns (SC1 and SC2) were acclimated with SE from a conventional wastewater treatment plant. This biological acclimation process was continued until both columns stabilized with respect to DOC reduction. The average influent DOC concentration during the acclimation period was 15.7 ± 1.7 mg/L and the effluent DOC was 12.5 ± 1.7 mg/L and 12.4 ± 1.6 mg/L for SC1 and SC2, respectively. On average DOC removal of about 20% was obtained in both soil columns at the end of the acclimation period (40-day).

The concentration of DOC in SE varied from 11 to 20 mg/L and the DOC in the DCW varied from 14 to 21 mg/L during the period of the study. DCW had a relatively higher SUVA value (3.22 L/mg-m) as compared to the SE (2.68 L/mg-m), indicating that the dissolved organic matter (DOM) in the DCW was more aromatic than the DOM in the SE. After both columns reached steady state with respect to DOC reduction, DCW with SE (1:1 ratio) and DCW were introduced into SC1 and SC2, respectively. Under steady state condition, the DOC concentration in the influent was reduced from 20.1 mg/L to 16.0 mg/L and from 15.1 mg/L to 12.6 mg/L in SC1 at a HLR of 2.8 m/day and 1.4 m/day respectively, resulting in corresponding DOC removal efficiencies of 20% and 17 %. However, in SC2 fed with DCW the DOC was reduced from 19.2 mg/L to 16.8 mg/L and from 17.4 mg/L to 15.6 mg/L at a HLR of 2.8 m/day and 1.4 m/day respectively, resulting in corresponding DOC removal efficiencies of 13% and 10%. Residence times for SC1 and SC2 were 4 days and 8 days, respectively. The removal of bulk organic matter in both SC1 and SC2 did not significantly change between the residence times of 4 days and 8 days. In addition, tracer study using NaCl was also carried out for columns studies to confirm the calculated residence times. A typical hydraulic residence time (travelling time) during BF is usually a month or more, and the range of HLR tested in this study may not be sufficient to observe its impact.

The impact of EfOM on the fate of bulk organic matter during soil passage was determined by comparing transformation of bulk organic matter in filtrates. At a HLR of 1.4 m/day, increasing DOC removals along the depth of SC1 and SC2 were observed. SC1 showed higher removal efficiency of DOC compared to SC2 because EfOM consists of the non-humic components (e.g., proteins or polysaccharides) that can be easily removed over short infiltration time. Thus, an increase of SUVA by 0.2 L/mg-m in SC1 reflects a preferential removal of non-humic compounds (aliphatic organic compounds) from EfOM over humic substances (aromatic carbon compounds) which were mainly present in DCW. Preferential removal of non-aromatic carbon was also observed during short travel times in the subsurface in a previous study (Amy and Drews, 2007). DCW showed higher aromaticity (SUVA) compared to that of typical surface waters used for drinking water resources. In the column experiment, a small fraction of humic substances from DCW was removed and most of organic fractions consisted of refractory compounds. The fate of each classification of organic matter in SC1 and SC2 is elaborated below under the section LC-OCD/OND measurements.

Biomass measurement

Figure 3.3 shows the ATP concentrations originating from the biomass associated with the sand, and DOC and dissolved oxygen (DO) concentrations in the water phase along the columns at different depths after 4 months of continuous operation. About 50% of total DOC removal and 64 to 70% of total DO reduction was observed in the top 50 cm layer of the soil columns under oxic conditions (Figure 3.3a and Figure 3.3c). The trends of ATP concentrations along the columns were very similar to that of the DOC and the DO concentrations under oxic conditions. The ATP concentrations in the first 5 cm layer was slightly higher in SC1 (188 ng ATP/cm^3) than in SC2 (166 ng ATP/cm^3). A higher concentration of ATP in SC1 reflects the influence of EfOM in the source water that has higher content of BDOC than the source water of SC2. The concentration of ATP in SC1 and SC2 was higher than the concentrations of biomass associated with a top layer (2-10 cm) of slow sand filters from drinking water treatment plants in the Netherlands (18-93 ng ATP/cm^3) (Magic-Knezev and van der Kooij 2004). This may be explained by the low BDOC concentration in influent and relatively higher HLR of a slow sand filter in a drinking water treatment plant. The ATP concentrations of the biomass associated with sand showed a good correlation with DOC reduction, and it is suggested that the DOC reduction could be used as an indicator of soil biomass. HPC was also carried out to enumerate the number of cultivable heterotrophic bacteria associated with sand from SC1. Cultivable bacteria are commonly a minor fraction of bacterial communities, and HPC cannot elucidate entire biomass activity (Vale et al., 2005). However, in this study, ATP concentrations were fairly well correlated to the HPC data (Figure 3.4). We observed a positive correlation between DOC removal and corresponding biomass indicator measurements as determined with both the ATP concentrations and the HPC values.

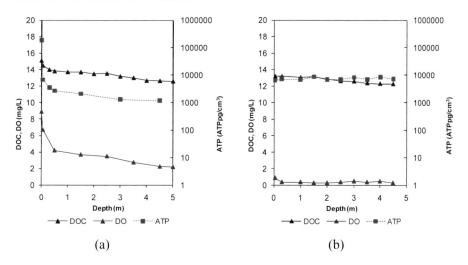

(a)   (b)

58

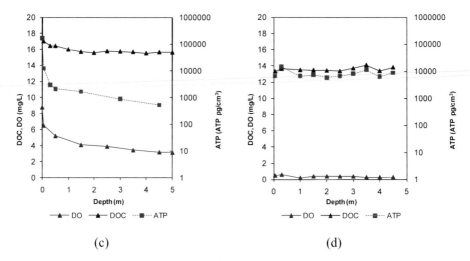

(c)　　　　　　　　　　　　　　　　(d)

Figure 3.3 ATP, DO and DOC profiles for SC1 (a) and SC2 (c) under oxic conditions, SC3 (b) and SC4 (d) under anoxic conditions (HLR: 1.4 m/day)

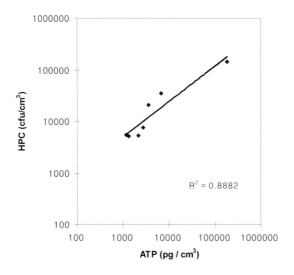

Figure 3.4 Correlation between ATP concentrations and HPC measurements at different depths of SC1 fed with a mixture of DCW and SE (1:1)

F-EEM

An F-EEM spectrum shows fluorescence intensity (FI) peaks at known wavelengths such that a FI peak at higher values of excitation and emission wavelengths corresponds to humic-like organic matter whereas a FI peak at lower values of excitation and emission wavelengths corresponds to protein-like organic matter (Amy and Drews, 2007). Figure 3.5 shows F-EEM spectra of influents and effluents of SC1 and SC2 at a HLR of 1.4 m/day (i.e., adjusted to ambient DOC). Samples from SC1 and SC2 showed no protein-like peak which usually appears in the excitation range from 250 to 280 nm and emission range from 280 to 350 nm. In activated sludge systems, bacteria produce EPS (extracellular polymeric substances) or

SMPs which play an important role in forming sludge flocs. The main components of EPS are proteins (up to 60%) and polysaccharides (40-95%) (Felmming and Wingender, 2001). In this study, most of the biopolymers in SE were polysaccharides which was supported by UV detection in LC-OCD measurement and explained below under the section of LC-OCD/OND. Polysaccharides are some of the most ubiquitous components in wastewater effluents (Lee et al., 2006).

Fluorescence wavelength differences could be interpreted as derived from NOM of different ages, origins and therefore different extents of degradation (Baker and Lamont-Black, 2001). In F-EEM spectra of SC1 and SC2, changes in locations of peaks between influent and effluent samples were not observed. However, changes (reductions) in FI were observed for all samples. These findings are due to the reduction in humic-like substances. Figure 3.6 shows the differential spectra between influent and effluent of SC1 and SC2. The spectrum of each effluent from SC1 and SC2 was subtracted from the influent spectrum SC1 and SC2. Humic-like EfOM and NOM in SC1 appears to be reduced more compared to that in SC2 which only consists of humic-like NOM. The humic components of EfOM was observed to be more biodegradable, however, a significant diminishment of the spectrum was not observed.

An attempt was made to use a quantifiable parameter such as a fluorescence ratio (FR) to assess the influence of SE on surface water. The FR of emission intensities at 450 to 500 nm at an excitation of 370 nm was found to be suggestive of either terrestrial-based (i.e., allochthonous) or algae- and bacteria-based (i.e., autochthonous) origins for the DOC (Donahue et al., 1998; McKnight et al., 2001). A FR value greater than 1.8 is correlated with DOC from autochthonous and a FR value less than 1.5 is more indicative of DOC derived from allchthonous. FR values in SC1 and SC2 samples were under 1.5 and considered as allochthonous. The FR value of SE was little higher that of DCW because of the influence of SE which contains SMPs responsible for the higher FR value. However, FR ratios of both samples were lower than 1.5 and there was no significant difference between DCW and SE (SE 1.4 and DCW 1.2); this may due to the high efficiency of the wastewater treatment plant in removing biodegradable organics and leaving only refractory humic-like compounds behind.

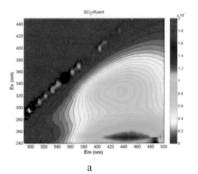

a

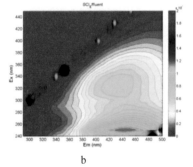

b

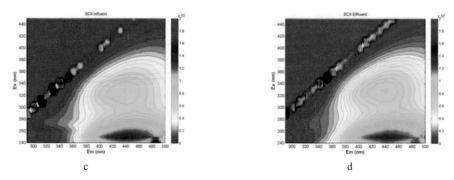

c   d

Figure 3.5 F-EEM spectra: (a) SC1 influent (top, left), (b) SC1 effluent (top, right), (c) SC2 influent and (d) SC2 effluent

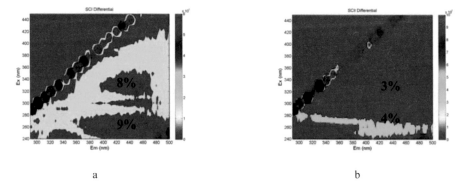

a   b

Figure 3.6 Differential F-EEM spectra (a) the SC1 effluent spectrum is subtracted from its influent spectrum, (b) the SC2 effluent spectrum is subtracted from its influent spectrum

LC-OCD/OND

LC-OCD/OND analysis of the samples from SC1 and SC2 were conducted, and the results are shown in Figures 3.7 and 3.8. LC-OCD/OND chromatograms showed a small fraction of organic matter in the range of biopolymers which is believed to be polysaccharides in influents from SC1 and SC2 because the absorbing peak from LC-UVA$_{254}$ did not appear, and theses fractions would also have appeared during F-EEM analysis if they were protein-like organic matter. LC-OCD/OND showed an almost complete removal of polysaccharides (high MW). SMPs in EfOM usually occurred across a wide range of molecular weights (MWs) (<0.5 to >50 kDa) according to the previous study (Barker and Stuckey, 1999). The biodegradation of different MW fractions in SEs showed that generally the high MW material was more readily degradable under oxic condition and the low MW was readily degraded anaerobically (Barker et al., 1999). Both soil columns SC1 and SC2 were operated under oxic conditions. Therefore, it was favorable for removal of high MW SMPs such as polysaccharides. This result is consistent with results from LC-OCD measurements at a bank filtration site at Lake Tegel (Berlin, Germany) in that only the fraction of polysaccharides shows a better removal under oxic conditions compared that of anoxic conditions (Jekel and Grünheid, 2005). Furthermore, the preferential removal of high MW (i.e., biopolymers) DOC in infiltration plays an important role in transformation of organic matter. Gerlach and Gimbel (1999) showed that humic substances with higher MWs are more favourably adsorbed onto soil and subsequently removed through microbial degradation to prevent the accumulation of soil organic matter in BF. In contrast to these results, the study done by Selenka and Hack (1995) concluded that biodegradation and sorption mechanisms equally removed DOC over the whole molecular size range. In the case of the wastewater effluent-impacted surface water, the transformation of organic matter may exhibit a different trend. However, further study is required to investigate the fate of EfOM (SMPs) produced from different types of biological wastewater treatment processes and redox conditions for a comprehensive understanding of EfOM during BF.

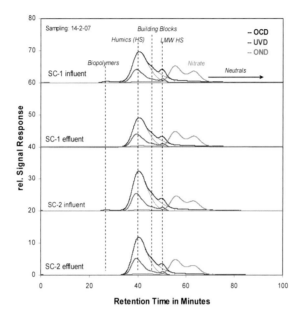

Figure 3.7 LC-OCD/OND chromatogram for SC1 (Delft canal water and wastewater effluent 1:1) and SC2 (Delft canal water) under oxic conditions

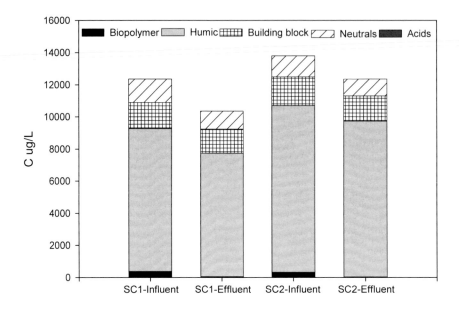

Figure 3.8 Change in organic matter fractions (biopolymer, humic substances, building blocks, neutrals and low MW acids) for SC1 and SC2 during soil passage under oxic conditions determined by LC-OCD

Table 3.4 Summary of organic matter fractions (biopolymer, humic substances, building blocks, neutrals and low MW acids)

Sample	Biopolymer (ug/L)	Humic substances (ug/L)	Building blocks (ug/L)	Neutrals (ug/L)	Low MW acids (ug/L)
SC1-Influent	374	8898	1620	1470	0
SC1-Effluent	50	7684	1512	1110	0
SC2-Influent	316	10388	1788	1308	0
SC2-Effluent	32	9702	1564	1052	0

3.3.2 Bulk organic matter characteristics-The River Meuse (SC3 and SC4)

DOC and DO

Two 5-meter long sand columns were used to investigate impacts of SE on BF performance and to get insight into the role of EfOM in SE on PhACs removal. The river Meuse (MR) and a mixture of MR and SE (1:1) were used for SC3 and SC4, respectively. The HLR was 1.4 m/day under oxic conditions. Table 3.5 shows pH, DOC, BDOC and SUVA values for the

SC3 and the SC4. For SC4, SUVA increased as a result of biodegradation of aliphatic organic matter.

Table 3.5 Characteristics of influent and effluent – SC3 and SC4

	Sample	pH	DOC (mg/L)	BDOC (mg/L)	SUVA (L/mg-m)
SC3 (MR)	Influent	7.85	3.66		2.46
SC3 (MR)	Effluent	7.81	2.99	0.67	2.34
SC4 (MR+SE)	Influent	7.50	9.67		2.90
SC4 (MR+SE)	Effluent	7.99	6.43	3.24	3.27

F-EEM

F-EEM spectra were measured for SC3 and SC4. Table 3.6 shows the reduction of the peaks in F-EEM spectra (P1, P2 and P3) of SC3 and SC4. Wastewater effluent-impacted surface water consists of SMPs which originate from a biological wastewater treatment process, and the main components of SMPs in the EfOM are comprised of proteins (up to 60%) and polysaccharides (40-95%) (Felmming and Wingender 2001). As shown in Table 3.5, fluorescence intensities (FI) of P1, P2 and P3 gradually reduced along the passage of the column for SC3 and SC4. Reductions in FI of P3 at 2.5 and 5 meters for SC4 were greater than that of the SC3. Protein-like substances (SMPs) in SE (P3) appear to be more biodegradable, thus a significant reduction of the FI was observed in P3 for SC4. Moreover, under more reducing conditions (i.e., anoxic conditions), FI reductions for P1 and P2 appeared to be relatively low compared to that under oxic conditions, because of the slow biotransformation of organic matter containing fluorescence properties. Dyckmans et al. (2006) examined soil microbial activity under oxic and anoxic conditions by measuring adenylate and phospholipid fatty acid contents. A high level of microbial activity was observed under oxic conditions compared to that under anoxic conditions. However, under anoxic conditions, the reduction of FI in P3 was still observed for both SC3 and SC4.

Table 3.6 Reductions of fluorescence intensity for humic-like peaks (P1 and P2) and protein-like peak (P3) for SC3 and SC4

	P1 (%)	P2 (%)	P3 (%)
SC3 (Oxic)	33	19	42
SC4 (Oxic)	15	26	60
SC3 (Anoxic)	5	5	57
SC4 (Anoxic)	0	2.2	38

LC-OCD

Figure 3.9 and Table 3.7 show the LC-OCD results of SC3 (fed with MR) and SC4 (fed with MR+SE). Biopolymers defined by LC-OCD (MW>20,000 Da) in SC3 and SC4 were removed 55% and 91%, respectively. The biopolymer fraction in SC4 was removed significantly during the column study. This result was consistent with that of SC1 which was fed with DCW amended with SE (1:1). The biopolymer fraction in SC1 was preferentially removed during soil passage. According to previous studies, biopolymers were significantly removed during biofiltration, whereas removal efficiencies of humic were much lower (Halle et al., 2009; Maeng et al., 2008). Removal efficiencies of the humic fraction from SC3 and SC4 were 11% and 22%, respectively. Part of the humic fraction from SE which was used for SC4 had more biodegradable characteristics. As shown in Figure 3.9, a significant amount of protein-like substances was removed in wastewater effluent-impacted surface water compared to the humic-like substances. Further study is required to investigate the fate of EfOM produced from different types of biological processes because the composition of EfOM can vary under different conditions (e.g., different hydraulic retention time (HRT) and solid retention time (SRT)). For example, a membrane bioreactor (MBR) runs under high biomass and long SRT; EfOM from a MBR plant consequently consists of more biomass associated products as result of the biomass decay (i.e., refractory organic matter).

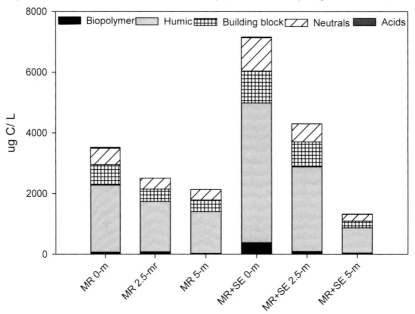

Figure 3.9 Change in organic matter fractions (biopolymer, humic substances, building blocks, neutrals and low MW acids) for MR (SC3) and MR+SE (SC4) during soil passage determined by LC-OCD

Table 3.7 Summary of organic matter fractions with respect to biopolymer, humic substances, building blocks, neutrals and low MW acids

Sample	Biopolymer (ug/L)	Humic substances (ug/L)	Building blocks (ug/L)	Neutrals (ug/L)	Low MW acids (ug/L)
SC3-Influent	63	2218	672	541	35
SC3-Effluent	26	1383	379	348	0
SC4-Influent	377	4610	1052	1092	25
SC4-Effluent	4	829	230	218	1

3.3.3 Effects of EfOM on the removal of pharmaceutically active compounds during BF

In this study, two sand column setups were used to compare the attenuation of 13 selected pharmaceuticals (see Table 3.1) in the river Meuse (SC3) and the river Meuse amended with SE (SC4). Table 3.8 shows removal efficiencies of selected PhACs from SC3 and SC4. Removal efficiencies of ibuprofen, fenoprofen, naproxen, ketoprofen, phenacetine, pentoxifylline and caffeine for SC4 (fed with MR+SE (1:1)) were similar to that of SC3 (fed with MR). However, gemfibrozil exhibited relatively low removal efficiency for SC4 (28%) compared to SC3 (97%) under oxic conditions. Diclofenac showed 76% and 15% removal efficiencies for SC3 and SC4, respectively. Also, bezafibrate also showed relatively low removal efficiency (49%) for SC4 compared to SC3 (97%). The low removal efficiencies was observed in wastewater effluent-impacted surface water for diclofenac, gemibrozil and bezafibrate under both oxic and anoxic conditions. These results implied that there were some impacts of EfOM on PhACs removal. From F-EEM and LC-OCD analyses, the biotransformation of DOM in wastewater effluent-impacted surface water was different than in surface water because EfOM contains SMPs which originate from a wastewater treatment plant. In other words, diclofenac, gemfibrozil and bezafibrate removals are negatively correlated to the EfOM concentration. This implies that the organic matter derived from SE (i.e., EfOM) diminished removal efficiencies of these compounds in some ways. This is a significantly important implication for water utilities where they use drinking water sources under the influence of wastewater effluent. In a previous study, the character of bulk organic carbon present in effluents affected the degradation of trace organic compounds during recharge operation (Rauch-Williams et al., 2010). Lim et al. (2008) showed that biotransformation rates of some PhACs (i.e., wastewater-derived contaminants) were different in microcosms containing different sources of biodegradable dissolved organic carbon (BDOC). They found out that BDOC derived from aquatic plants enhanced the removal of certain refractory compounds (e.g., gemfibrozil) as compared to BDOC derived from SE. In other words, they suggested that there were differences in microbial diversity and functionality among different water sources. However, in order to explain different removal efficiencies for some PhACs observed between wastewater effluent-impacted surface water and surface water, further investigations are necessary to define the biodiversity of microbial community in different water sources.

Active microbial biomass (AMB) associated with sand was determined by measuring ATP concentration for SC3 and SC4 columns. ATP concentrations at 0.1, 2.5 and 5 m depths of the SC3 column were 151, 20 and 4 ng ATP/cm^3, respectively. ATP concentrations for the SC4 column were 253, 94 and 9 ng ATP/cm^3 at 0.1, 2.5 and 5 m depth, respectively. AMB decreased with depth of the columns. Average concentrations of AMB and BDOC for SC4 (AMB: 58 ng ATP/cm^3, BDOC: 3.17 mg/l) were higher than those of SC3 (AMB: 28 ng ATP/cm^3, BDOC: 2.95 mg/L). However, the amount of AMB and BDOC did not show a positive correlation with the biotransformation for diclofenac, gemfibrozil and bezafibrate. This result does not mean the availability of BDOC is not important, but the characteristics of BDOC or biodiversity are also equally important to consider for some PhACs. There was more AMB in the column (SC4) fed with wastewater effluent-impacted effluent, however, AMB may consist of dominant species that are unable to biotransform diclofenac, gemfibrozil and bezafibrate. On the other hand, the physical adsorption or the degree of ionization of gemifibrozil and diclofenac on bioactive sand is interfered by the EfOM. Gemfibrozil and diclofenac remained as ionic species because their acid dissociation constants (pKa) are 4.7 and 4.2, respectively. The pH of the River Meuse and SE (pH 7.50 to

7.99) were higher than pK_a of gemfibroail (4.7) and Diclofenac (4.2). However, there were also other ionic compounds. For example, ibuprofen and fenoprofen remained as ionic compounds, but their removal efficiencies were similar and high for both wastewater effluent-impacted surface water and surface water. In this study, microorganisms from the river Meuse were able to biotransform gemifibrozil and diclofenac, while microorganisms in wastewater effluent-impacted surface water may have a number of dominant microorganisms which cannot produce enzymes to biotransform gemifibrozil and diclofenac. Further research is required to define complex microbial communities in surface water and a SE.

Figure 3.10 shows the biotransformation of selected PhACs at different depths (e.g., 0-m, 2.5-m and 5-m) from SC3 and SC4 under oxic condition. Samples took at different depths of columns represent as travel times in Figure 3.10. Most of the PhACs showed a first order reaction except gemfibrozil, diclofenac, clofibric acid and carbamazepine. Redox conditions in a feed container were changed from oxic to anoxic conditions using nitrogen gas (i.e., 24-hr continuous nitrogen gas purging). However, no significant difference was observed with respect to removal efficiencies of selected PhACs compounds between oxic and anoxic conditions (Table 3.8). Again, bezafibrate, gemifibrozil and diclofenac were removed greater for SC3 compared to SC4 under anoxic conditions, and carbamazepine showed a persistent behaviour under all conditions. Table 3.9 shows the summary of overall removal of total PhACs (i.e., Σ PhACs in effluent / Σ PhACs in influent) for SC3 and SC4. The overall removal of SC3 under oxic conditions was the highest followed by SC3 (anoxic), SC4 (oxic) and SC4 (anoxic).

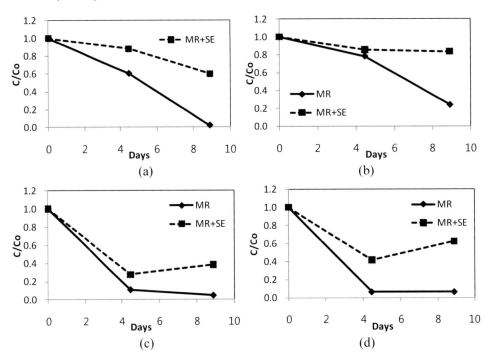

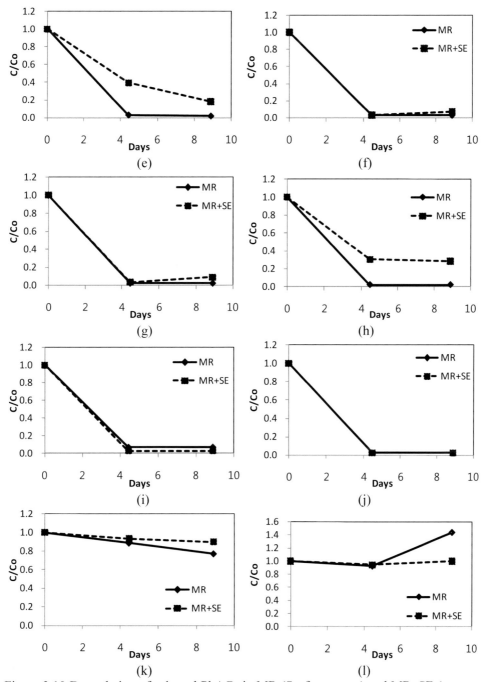

Figure 3.10 Degradation of selected PhACs in MR (Surface water) and MR+SE (wastewater effluent-dominated surface water) under oxic conditions: (a) gemfibrozil, (b) diclofenac, (c) bezafibrate, (d) fenoprofen, (e) ketoprofen, (f) naproxen, (g) ibuprofen, (h) pentoxifylline, (i) caffeine, (j) phenacetine, (k) clofibric acid, (l) carbamazepine

Table 3.8 Removal efficiency of PhACs for SC3 and SC4

	MR (SC3, Oxic)	MR+SE (SC4, Oxic)	MR (SC3, Anoxic)	MR+SE (SC4, Anoxic)
Gemfibrozil	97	28	98	12
Diclofenac	76	15	76	17
Ibuprofen	98	88	98	91
Fenoprofen	94	70	94	38
Bezafibrate	97	49	95	62
Ketoprofen	97	67	98	61
Naproxen	98	95	97	93
Clofibric acid	32	29	23	10
Carbamazepine	0	0	0	0
Phenacetine	98	95	98	98
Pentoxifylline	98	95	98	72
Paracetamol	98		96	
Caffeine	98	97	93	97

Table 3.9 Summary of overall removal (i.e., Σ PhACs in effluent / Σ PhACs in influent) of PhACs for SC3 and SC4

	SC3 MR (Oxic)	SC4 MR+SE (Oxic)	SC3 MR (Anoxic)	SC4 MR+SE (Anoxic)
Removal %	82	58	74	56

3.4. Conclusions

Based on the results obtained in this study, the following conclusions can be drawn:

- The characteristics of bulk organic matter in surface water (DCW) and wastewater effluent-impacted surface water were different. However, the residual organic matter characteristics after soil passage were similar and overlap each other.
- DCW had a relatively higher SUVA value (3.22 L/mg-m) as compared to SE (2.68 L/mg-m). This indicates the DOC compounds in DCW are more aromatic (humic-like) than the DOC compounds in the SE.
- The fluorescence analysis for both SC1 and SC2 filtrates revealed the reduction of humic like substances after soil passage was not significant. No protein-like substances was observed in the filtrates indicating that these components are easily removed during soil passage.
- LC-OCD/OND showed an almost complete removal of biopolymers believed to be polysaccharides, however, the other four fractions were not significantly removed.
- 50% of total DOC removal and 64 to 70% of total DO reduction were observed in the top 50 cm layer of the soil columns. This was presumably due to biodegradation of organic matter by the biomass associated with the sand which was determined by ATP concentrations and heterotrophic plate count. Good correlation of DOC removal with DO and biomass development was observed in the soil columns. High concentrations of

ATP in the first few centimeters of infiltration surface reflect the highest microbial activity in this part of the column which correlates with the extent of DOC reduction.

- Biodegradable organic matter (e.g., biopolymer) in EfOM, which originates from biological wastewater treatment processes, was effectively removed during soil passage.
- Most of the selected PhACs exhibited removal efficiencies greater than 90% in both wastewater effluent-impacted surface water and as well as surface water.
- Removal efficiencies of bezafibrate, diclofenac, and gemfibrozil were relatively low in wastewater effluent-impacted surface water which appears to have more biodegradable organic matter from EfOM. This result indicates that organic matter characteristics or microbial diversity affect the biotransformation of some recalcitrant PhACs.
- Carbamazepine and clofibric acid showed a persistent behavior and were not influenced by EfOM.
- The removal efficiencies of the selected PhACs under different redox conditions (i.e., oxic and anoxic conditions) were not significantly different in this study.
- The overall removal of selected PhACs was lower in wastewater effluent-impacted surface water compared to that of surface water under both oxic and anoxic conditions.
- Further study is required to define microorganisms responsible for biotransformation of some PhACs in surface water.

3.5. References

Amy, G. and Drews, J., 2007. Soil Aquifer Treatment (SAT) as Natural and Sustainable Wastewater Reclamation/Reuse Technology: Fate of Wastewater Effluent Organic Matter (EfOM) and Trace Organic Compounds. Environ Monit Assess, 129(1-3), 19-26.

Baker, A. and Lamont-Black, J., 2001. Fluorescence of dissolved organic mater as natural tracer of ground water. Ground Water, 39(5), 745-750.

Barker, D. J., Mannucchi, G. A., Salvi, S. M. L. and Stuckey, D. C., 1999. Characterisation of soluble residual chemical oxygen demand (COD) in anaerobic wastewater treatment effluents. Water Res., 33(11), 2499-2510.

Barker, D. J. and Stuckey, D. C., 1999. A review of soluble microbial products (SMP) in wastewater treatment systems. Water Res., 33(14), 3063-3082.

Coble, P.G., 1996. Characterization of marine and terrestrial DOM in seawater using excitation-emission matrix spectroscopy. Mar. Chem., 51(4), 325-346.

Donahue, W. F., Schindler, D. W., Page, S. J. and Stainton, M. P., 1998. Acid-Induced Changes in DOC Quality in an Experimental Whole-Lake Manipulation. Environ. Sci. and Technol., 32(19), 2954-2960.

Dyckmans J., Flessa H., Lipsk A., Potthoff M. and Beese F., 2006. Microbial biomass and activity under oxic and anoxic conditions as affected by nitrate additions. Journal of Plant Nutrition and Soil Science, 169, 108-115.

Felmming, H.-C. and Wingender, J., 2001. Relevance of microbial extracellular polymeric substances (EPSs) - Part I: Structural and ecological aspects. Wat. Sci. Tech., 43(6), 1-8.

Gerlach, M. and Gimbel, R., 1999. Influence of humic substance alteration during soil passage on their treatment behaviour. Wat. Sci. Tech., 40(9), 231-239.

Grünheid, S., Amy, G. and Jekel, M., 2005. Removal of bulk dissolved organic carbon (DOC) and trace organic compounds by bank filtration and artificial recharge. Water Res., 39(14), 3219.

Halle C., Huck P.M., Peldszus S., Haberkamp J. and Jekel M., 2009. Assessing the Performance of Biological Filtration As Pretreatment to Low Pressure Membranes for Drinking Water. Environ. Sci. Technol. 43, 3878-3884.

Heberer, T., Mechlinski, A., Fanck, B., Knappe, A., Massmann, G., Pekdeger, A. and Fritz, B., 2004. Field studies on the fate and transport of pharmaceutical residues in bank filtration. Ground Water Monit. R., 24(2), 70-77.

Henderson, R. K., Baker, A., Murphy, K. R., Hambly, A., Stuetz, R. M. and Khan, S. J. 2009. Fluorescence as a potential monitoring tool for recycled water systems: A review. Water Res. 43(4), 863-881.

Irmscher, R. and Teermann, I., 2002. Riverbank filtration for drinking water supply - a proven method, perfect to face today's challenge. Water Sci. Technol., 2(5-6), 1-8.

Jarusutthirak, C. and Amy, G., 2006. Role of soluble microbial products (SMP) in membrane foulding and flux decline. Environ. Sci. and Technol., 40(3), 969-974.

Jekel, M. and Gruenheid, S., 2005. Bank filtration and groundwater recharge for treatment of polluted surface waters. Wat. Sci. Tech., 5(5), 57-66.

Kim, S. D., Cho, J., Kim, I. S., Vanderford, B. J. and Snyder, S. A., 2007. Occurrence and removal of pharmaceuticals and endocrine disruptors in South Korean surface, drinking, and waste waters. Water Res., 41(5), 1013-1021.

Lee, S., Ang, W. S., and Elimelech, M., 2006. Fouling of reverse osmosis membranes by hydrophilic organic matter: implications for water reuse. Desalination, 187(1-3), 313-321.

Leenheer, J. A., and Croue, J.-P., 2003. Characterizing aquatic dissolved organic matter. Environ. Sci. and Technol., 37(1), 18A-26A.

Levine, A. D., Tchobanoglous, G., and Asano, T., 1985. Characterization of the size distribution of contaminants in wastewater: treatment and reuse implications. Journal WPCF, 57(7), 805-816.

Lim M.-H., Snyder S.A., Sedlak D.L., 2008. Use of biodegradable dissolved organic carbon (BDOC) to assess the potential for transformation of wastewater-derived contaminants in surface waters. Water Res. 42, 2943-2952.

Madden, J. C., Enoch, S. J., Hewitt, M., and Cronin, M. T. D., 2009. Pharmaceuticals in the environment: Good practice in predicting acute ecotoxicological effects. Toxicol. Lett., 185(2), 85-101.

Maeng S.K., Sharma S.K., Magic-Knezev A. and Amy, G.L., 2008. Fate of effluent organic matter (EfOM) and natural organic matter (NOM) through riverbank filtration. Water Sci. Technol. 57,1999–2007.

Magic-Knezev, A. and van der Kooij, D., 2004. Optimisation and significance of ATP analysis for measuring active biomass in granular activated carbon filters used in water treatment. Water Res., 38(18), 3971-3979.

Massmann, G., Greskowiak, J., Dünnbier, U. and Zuehlke, S., 2006. The impact of variable temperatures on the redox conditions and the behavior of pharmaceutical residues during artificial recharge. J. Hydrol., 328, 141-156.

Massmann, G., Dunnbier, U., Heberer, T. and Taute, T., 2008. Behaviour and redox sensitivity of pharmaceutical residues during bank filtration - Investigation of residues of phenazone-type analgesics. Chemosphere, 71(8), 1476-1485.

Mechlinski, A. and Heberer, T., 2005. Fate and transport of pharmaceutical residues during bank filtration. In: ISMAR 2005, Berlin, 542-547.

McKnight, D. M., Boyer, E. W., Doran, P. T., Westerhoff, P. K., Kulbe, T. and Anderson., D. T., 2001. Spectrofluorometric characterization of aquatic fulvic acid for determination of precursor organic material and general structural properties. Limnol. Oceanorg., 46(1), 38-48.

Mompelat, S., LeBot, B. and Thomas, O., 2009. Occurrence and fate of pharmaceutical products and by-products, from resource to drinking water. Environment International, 35, 803-814.

Oades, J. M. and Jenkinson, D. S., 1979. Adenosine triphosphate content of the soil microbial biomass. Soil Biology and Biochemistry, 11(2), 201-204.

Rauch-Williams, T. and Drewes, J. E., 2005. Quantifying biological organic removal in groundwater recharge systems." J. Environ. Eng., 131(6), 909-923.

Rauch-Williams, T., Hoppe-Jones, C. and Drewes J. E., 2010. The role of organic matter in the removal of emerging trace organic chemicals during managed aquifer recharge. Water Res. 44(2), 449-460.

Sacher, F., Ehmann, M., Gabriel, S., Graf, C. and Brauch, H.-J., 2008. Pharmaceutical residues in the river Rhine—results of a one-decade monitoring programme. J. Environ. Monit. 10, 664-670.

Schmidt, C. K., Lange, F. T. and Brauch, H. J., 2007. Characteristics and evaluation of natural attenuation processes for organic micropollutant removal during riverbank filtration. In: Regional IWA conference on groundwater management in the Danube River Basin and other large River Basins, 7-9 June 2007, Belgrade, Serbia, 231-236.

Selenka, F. and Hack, A., 1995. Transport, Umsetzung und mikrobieller Abbau natürlicher und anthropogener organischer Substanzen im Grundwasser bei Uferfiltration und kunstlicher Grundwasseranreicherung, VCH, Weinheim.

USEPA, 2003. National Primary Regulations: Long Term 2 Enhanced Surface Water Treatment Rule, Proposed rule, (June 30, 2003), 40CFR Part 141 and 142, Washington, D.C.

Vale, M., Nguyen, C., Dambrine, E. and Dupouey, J. L., 2005. "Microbial activity in the rhizosphere soil of six herbaceous species cultivated in a greenhouse is correlated with shoot biomass and root C concentrations." Soil Biology and Biochemistry, 37(12), 2329-2333.

Velten, S., Hammes, F., Boller, M. and Egli, T., 2007. Rapid and direct estimation of active biomass on granular activated carbon through adenosine tri-phosphate (ATP) determination. Water Res., 41(9), 1973-1983.

Chapter 4
FATE OF ENDOCRINE DISRUPTING COMPOUNDS DURING BANK FILTRATION

Summary

The objective of this study was to determine the fate of estrogen compounds during bank filtration. Laboratory-scale batch and soil columns experiments were conducted to determine factors influencing the removal of estrogen compounds (estrone, 17β-estradiol and 17α-ethinylestradiol) during soil passage and determine. Biotic and abiotic batch experiments were also employed to investigate the role of microbial activity in the removal. Moreover, batch experiments were also conducted under different redox conditions to investigate the impact of redox conditions on the removal of estrogen compounds. Both batch and soil column studies showed that adsorption and biodegradation are the two important removal mechanisms for estrone, 17β-estradiol and 17α-ethinylestradiol, of which adsorption was the important removal mechanism. 17β-estradiol and 17α-ethinylestradiol were removed 99% and 96%, respectively, in batch experiments under oxic conditions (hydraulic retention time: 5 days). Microbial activity associated with the soil (sand) and redox conditions did not show any significant effects on the removal of 17β-estradiol. However, 17α-ethinylestradiol removals varied from 64% to 87% in soil columns fed with different sources of water. Estrogenic activity remaining under oxic conditions (13 ng estradiol-equivalents/L) was significantly lower than that of under anoxic conditions (97 ng estradiol-equivalents/L).

4.1. Introduction

The use of organic chemicals has been increasing over the last four decades, and consequently, their presenceit causes abnormalities in the aquatic environment (Blaber, 1970; Gomes and Lester, 2003; Smith, 1971). With rapid development in technology and instrumentation, researchers are able to measure emerging organic micropollutants (OMPs) more accurately, and these emerging contaminants can now be measured in the range of parts per trillion (ppt). OMPs often include personal care products (PCPs), endocrine disrupting compounds (EDCs) and pharmaceutically active compounds (PhACs). Moreover, there is an increasing concern about the presence of EDCs in the aquatic environment (Shappel, 2006). EDCs have been recognized as a new category of environmental contaminants that interrupt the function(s) of endocrine systems (Colborn and Clement, 1992).

Many EDCs exhibit neutral and hydrophobic characteristics, and are favorably absorbed onto particulates. Therefore, most EDCs are often concentrated in suspended solids or sediment versus the aqueous phase, and the intrusion of EDCs into ground water is minimized by these characteristics. Ground waters are less influenced by EDCs compared to surface waters. However, sediments can be dynamic under seasonal variations. During times of flooding, the increased flow of a river may cause scouring of riverbed layer (i.e., increased porosity) that leads to possible intrusion of EDCs. Therefore, the degradation of bound EDCs is important to investigate, and it is dependent on numerous factors, including: redox conditions, temperature, dissolved organic matter and pH. Figure 4.1 shows the behavior of EDCs in the receiving aquatic environment and their sources.

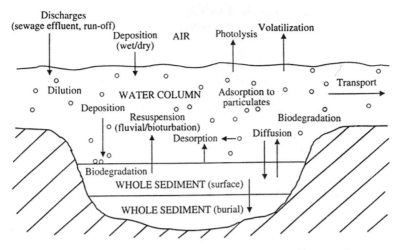

Source: Gomes et al. (2003)

Figure 4.1 Sources and behavior of EDCs in the receiving aquatic environment.

Among the many EDCs, estrogens such as estrone (E1), 17β-estradiol (E2) and 17α-ethinylestradiol (EE2) showed the most estrogenic activity, and alkylphenols and their ethoxylates showed less estrogenic activity than that of estrogens (Gomes and Lester, 2003). Moreover, E1, E2 and EE2 possess estrogenic potency 10,000 to 100,000 times higher than exogenous EDCs such as organochlorine aromatic compounds (Cargouët et al., 2004; Gomes and Lester, 2003; Hanselman et al., 2003). Natural estrogens (E1 and E2) and synthetic estrogens (EE2) have received most of the scientific attention and are classified as EDCs (Birkett., 2003). Wastewater treatment plants receive a large variety of EDCs but cannot always effectively remove these compounds with conventional wastewater treatment technologies before discharging effluent into receiving water bodies or land. Recently, several studies showed the presence of estrogens in surface waters, wastewater and treated wastewater in different parts of the world (Carballa et al., 2004; Cargouët et al., 2004; Hintemann et al., 2006; Lishman et al., 2006; Ma et al., 2007; Nakada et al., 2005; Sarmah et al., 2006). Ternes et al. (1999) showed the frequent presence of E1 and E2 in effluents discharged from German and Canadian sewage treatment plants over ranges of ng/L, with a maximum concentration of 70 ng/L for estrone. A number of studies have reported that the feminization of male aquatic species in receiving waters mainly originated from the effluents from wastewater treatment plants, and surface runoff from agricultural activities and municipal biosolids (Khanal et al., 2006). In addition, this is of concern for water utilities where their raw water is strongly influenced by wastewater effluent. Therefore, there is a possibility for residual EDCs in drinking water sources that could adversely impact human health. However, further studies are needed to determine the effects of EDC concentrations in drinking water sources on human health.

Natural estrogens (E2 and E1) have a similar molecular framework, which is composed of four rings; a phenol, two cyclo hexanes and a cyclo-pentane. The difference in compound lies only in the D-ring configuration at positions C16 and C17 (Khanal et al., 2006). E2 is transformed to E1 under oxic conditions but the transformation rate varies according to the availability of electron acceptors and properties of the estrogens compound (Czajka and Londry, 2006). Physicochemical properties of E1, E2 and EE2 are shown in the Table 4.1 .

Table 4.1 Physiochemical properties of steroid estrogens

	Estrone	17β-Estradiol	17α-Ethinylestradiol
Structure			
Formula	$C_{18}H_{22}O_2$	$C_{18}H_{24}O_2$	$C_{20}H_{24}O_2$
Vapor pressure (kPa)	0.1 – 0.2	1	1 - 2
Solubility in water at 20°C	0.8 – 12.4	5.4 – 13.3	3.4 – 4
Octanol-water partitioning coefficients (log K_{ow})	3.43	3.43	4.15
Molecular weight g/mol	270.37	272.38	296.4
Natural estrogen	YES	YES	NO (synthetic)
Removal mechanism	Sorption and subsequent biodegradation	Sorption and subsequent biodegradation	Sorption and subsequent biodegradation
Type of compound	Moderately hydrophobic and moderately soluble in water	Moderately hydrophobic and moderately soluble in water	Hydrophobic and poorly soluble in water
Acronyms	E1	E2	EE2

Source: Modified and reproduced from Birkett (2003)

Estrogen compounds have a hydrophobic characteristic, which is favorable to their adsorption during wastewater treatment processes or bank filtration (BF). Estrogens such as E1, E2 and EE2 have high octanol-water partition coefficients (K_{ow}). K_{ow} is a (log) concentration ratio at equilibrium of organic compounds partitioning between octanol and water phases. Therefore, if a compound partitions into octanol, it is expected to easily adsorb onto the sediment or granular activated carbon (GAC). Values of the adsorption capacity coefficient (K_f) of different types of soil vary from 4 (sand) to as high as 667 (LaDelle silt loam). K_f is an important parameter because it is strongly correlated to the organic content (fraction organic carbon, f_{OC}) of the sorbent, as pure sand, silt, and clay contain very low organic matter; whereas LaDelle silt loam, which contains a high organic matter content, was found to be a strong adsorbent of free estrogens (Khanal et al., 2006). However, in our study, different types of soil were not used to investigate the impact of K_f on the removal of estrogen compounds. This study focused on the microbial activity associated with bio-acclimated sand to determine the role of biodegradation in the removal of estrogen compounds.

The biodegradation of EDCs from water, sediments and soils is expected to occur as a result of a combination of physical sorption and binding on biomass. Published studies showed that natural estrogens (E1 and E2) in wastewater treatment plants or batch experiments using municipal sludge were largely degraded biologically (Andersen et al., 2003; Khanal et al., 2006; Shappel, 2006; Suzuki and Maruyama, 2006). The removal mechanism of the estrogens during soil infiltration was observed to be adsorption onto the soil and subsequent additional attenuation by biodegradation. The degradation of free estrogens occurred mainly through a biotic route, whereas under abiotic conditions, the estrogen level fairly remained constant at an initial estrogen level in a column study (Mansell et al., 2004; Ying et al., 2003). Moreover, the removal of transformation products should be considered beyond the attenuation of the parent compound (e.g., E2) because the transformation products from E2 oxidation still possess estrogenic activity. It is important to note that estrogenic activity from transformation products must be considered to accurately estimate the removal of estrogen compounds. Thus, 14C-labeled E2 compound was used to demonstrate its fate during an activated sludge process (i.e., conventional wastewater treatment process), and the activated sludge process was capable of mineralizing 70 to 80% of E2 to carbon dioxide in 24 h (Layton et al., 2000). The degradation pathway of E2 with microbial enzyme and industrial catalyst is illustrated in Figure 4.2 (Khanal et al., 2006). E2 was oxidized from the cyclo-pentane ring D at C17 into E1 during enzymatic degradation and then further degraded into metabolite X1 and finally to carbon dioxide through a tricarboxylic acid (TCA) cycle.

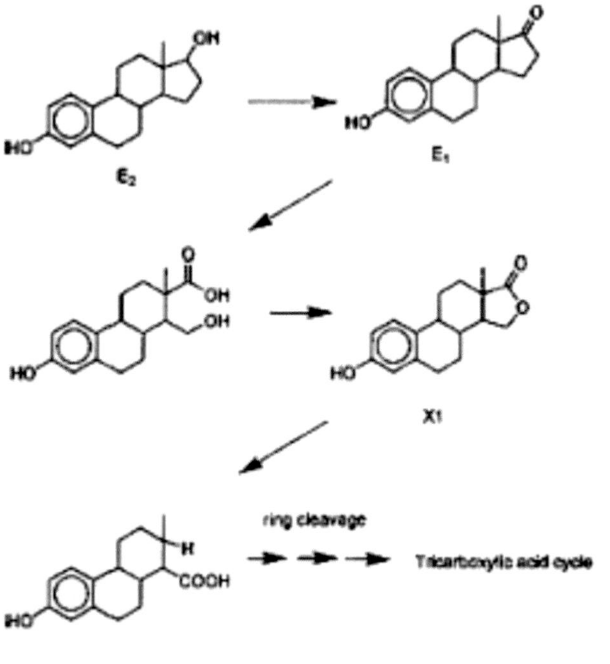

Source: Khanal et al. (2006)

Figure 4.2 Pathway of 17β-estradiol (E2) degradation

Proper understanding and analysis of the fate of E2, E1 and EE2 during soil passage is essential to optimise their removals during BF. It is equally important to investigate factors influencing the removal of the estrogen compounds during BF for their proper design and operation. The main goal of this particular study was to evaluate the fate of estrogen compounds during BF. The specific objectives to achieve this goal were:

(i) To investigate the fate of E2, E1 and EE2 during BF using batch and soil column studies

(ii) To investigate the fate of estrogens during BF under different redox conditions

(iii) To determine the relative performance of a biodegradation and adsorption for the removal of E1, E2 and EE2

(iv) To investigate the feasibility of monitoring E2 and EE2 using solid phase extraction followed by fluorescence

4.2. Materials and methods

Batch and soil column studies were conducted to investigate the fate of estrogen compounds during BF.

4.2.1. Abiotic experiment

Batch reactors were first used to determine the concentration of sodium azide required for inactivating the microbial activity of microorganisms associated with sand (i.e., establishing abiotic conditions). Oxic conditions were maintained during the experiments, and Delft canal water (DCW) and secondary effluent (SE) from Hoek van Holland wastewater treatment plant (Hoek van Holland, The Netherlands) were used as influents. Three different concentrations (2 mM, 10 mM and 20 mM) of sodium azide were tested, and Table 4.2 shows a summary of the experimental set-up for this experiment.

Table 4.2 Batch reactor set-up for abiotic experiment

Sodium azide concentration	Influents	Redox conditions	Silica sand (0.8-1.25 mm)
2 mM	DCW + SE (1:1 ratio)	Oxic	Acclimated sand
10 mM	DCW + SE (1:1 ratio)	Oxic	Acclimated sand
20 mM	DCW + SE (1:1 ratio)	Oxic	Acclimated sand
Blank (0 mM)	DCW + SE (1:1 ratio)	Oxic	Acclimated sand

4.2.2. Factors affecting the removals of E2, E1 and EE2

Batch experiments were conducted to investigate factors influencing E2, E1 and EE2 removals during BF. Batch reactor set-ups were divided into two identical (parallel) set-ups because there was a high interference between EE2 and E2 measurements using enzyme-linked immunosorbent assay (ELISA) kits. Therefore, E2 and E1 were carried out in same batch reactors, and EE2 tests were conducted separately. 5 and 7 batch reactors were carried under biotic and abiotic conditions (oxic conditions), respectively. The same numbers of the batch reactors were also conducted under anoxic conditions. Table 4.3 shows a summary of the batch reactor set-ups.

Table 4.3 Summary of batch reactor set-up for E1, E2 and EE2

Batch reactor set-up (duplicate)	Redox conditions / Biotic or abiotic conditions
Autoclaved Tap Water (ACTW)	Oxic / Abiotic
DCW and SE (1:1) + Sodium azide	Oxic / Abiotic
DCW and SE (1:1)	Oxic / Biotic
Fresh sand + ACTW	Oxic / Abiotic
DCW and SE (1:1)	Oxic / Biotic
Fresh sand + DCW and SE (1:1)	Oxic / Biotic
Fresh sand + DCW and SE (1:1) + Sodium azide	Oxic / Abiotic
Acclimated sand + DCW and SE (1:1) + Sodium azide	Oxic / Abiotic
Acclimated sand + ACTW + Sodium azide	Oxic / Abiotic
Acclimated sand + ACTW	Oxic / Biotic
Acclimated sand + DCW and SE (1:1)	Oxic / Biotic
Acclimated sand + DCW and SE (1:1) + Sodium Azide	Oxic / Abiotic

4.2.3. Soil column study

The fate of estrogen compounds during BF was investigated by conducting laboratory-scale soil column studies. Silica sand (0.8 to 1.25 mm), (bio)acclimated for 60 days using secondary effluent, was used in 300 mm long columns comprised of inner and outer diameters (50 mm inner diameter, XK50/30, Amersham Pharmacia Biotech, Sweden). The inner part was packed with silica sand, while the outer one was used to control the prevailing ambient temperature by flowing water from a chillier. The columns were kept in a dark room to minimize effects from sunlight, and empty bed contact time (EBCT) was 11 hours.

4.2.4. E2, E1 and EE2 analyses by enzyme-linked immunosorbent assay (ELISA)

Estrogens were measured using ELISA kits which are based on a competitive reaction where enzyme labeled standard E1 (E2 or EE2) competes with free E1 (E2 or EE2) in a sample for binding to a specific monoclonal antibody immobilized to the surface of a microplate. The amount of labeled E1 (E2 or EE2) bound to the antibody is determined using a microplate reader at 450 nm. The color intensity is measured at 450 nm and allows measuring the concentration of E1, E2 and EE2. Standard solutions of E1, E2 and EE2 supplied with the ELISA kit were used for developing calibration curves of E2, E1 and EE2 (Japan EnviroChemicals Ltd.). A detailed description of methods used for ELISA is explained in the study done by Suzuki and Maruyama (2006).

4.2.5. Biomass measurement

Adenosine triphosphate (ATP) was measured to determine active biomass concentration on the sand in soil columns. A detailed description of methods used for ATP measurements is explained in the previous chapter (3.2.4).

4.2.6. Estrogenicity assays

A commercially available biosensor, the Estrogen Responsive Chemically Activated LUciferase eXpression (ER-CALUX) assay, was carried out by BioDetection Systems b.v. (Amsterdam, The Netherlands) to determine the estrogenic activity in a water sample. ER-CALUX was developed using the T47D human breast adenocarcinoma cell engineered to express an estrogen receptor (luiferase). The luciferase will luminesce (i.e., amount of luciferase production) when exposed to a chemical (e.g., estrogen compounds). The light emission or bioluminescence can bequantitatively measured using a luminometer. Results are expressed as ng estradiol-equivalent (EEQ) / l of water. More information on the ER-CALUX protocol is available in Legler et al. (2002).

4.2.7. Analytical methods for several parameters

Organic matter in all samples was characterized within 3 days after sample collection and stored at 4 °C after 0.45 μm filtration (Whatman, Dassel, Germany) to prevent biodegradation of organic matter. The concentration of bulk organic matter was determined as DOC by a total organic carbon analyzer (Shimadzu TOC-V$_{CPN}$). The characteristics of bulk organic matter were elucidated by various analytical methods including fluorescence excitation-emission matrix (F-EEM). In F-EEM analysis, all samples were adjusted to a pH 2 by diluting samples to 1 mg/L of DOC with 0.01 N KCl due to the fluorophore interferences by metals, and measured by a FluoroMax-3 spectrofluorometer (HORIBA Jobin Yvon, Edison, NJ, USA).

4.3. Results and discussion

4.3.1. Influent characteristics

A mixture of SE and DCW (1:1 ratio) was used as influent for batch reactors and soil columns. All samples were filtered with 0.45 μm polyvinylidene fluoride (PVDF) membranes and stored in a cold room at 4°C. Influent characteristics are presented in Table 4.4. Specific UV absorbance (SUVA) is the ratio between DOC and UVA at 254 nm, and shows the aromaticity or humic content of the bulk organic matter. Background concentrations of E1, E2 and EE2 in SE and DCW were below the limit of ELISA quantification (50 ng/L for E1, E2 and EE2).

Table 4.4 The characteristics of influent used for batch and soil column experiment

Parameters	Unit	Delft canal water (DCW)	Secondary effluent (SE)
pH	-	7.2	7.82
EC	μc/cm	1257	1000
DOC	mg/L	17.4	12.3
UV$_{254}$	cm^{-1}	0.5	0.4
SUVA	L/mg-m	3.2	3.2
NH$_4$-N	mg/L	0.2	0.1
NO$_3$-N	mg/L	2.2	1.8
PO$_4$-P	mg/L	1.1	0.3
SO$_4^{2-}$	mg/L	74.5	97.7

4.3.2. Acclimation of sand in batch reactors and soil columns

For batch experiments, batch reactors were prepared as follows: 100 g of clean dry sand of size 0.8 - 1.25 mm diameter was used and immersed in DCW and SE (1:1) up to 400 mL (working volume). All batch reactors were kept on a shaker and rotated at 100 rpm. The acclimation period was more than 2 months until the batch reactors stabilized with respect to DOC removal. During the acclimation period, DOC and UV_{254} from influent and effluent samples were continuously monitored, and the HRT of the batch reactor was 5 days. Average DOC concentrations of influent and effluent from batch reactors after the acclimation period were 12.3 ± 4.8 and 11.1 ± 4.5 mg/L, respectively.

Three soil columns (SC1, SC2 and SC3) were fed with a mixture of DCW and SE. Again before introducing estrogen standards; it took about 2 months (acclimation period) to stabilize DOC removal. Influent and effluent DOC concentrations were continuously monitored during this period. Oxic conditions were maintained by continuous aeration in a feed tank. Figure 4.3 shows the variation of DOC concentrations in influent and effluent samples during the acclimation period while Figure 4.4 represents a normalized plot which shows the extent of DOC removal during the acclimation period. The average DOC concentration for influent was 14.5 ± 2.9 mg/L. Effluent samples from SC1, SC2 and SC3 had DOC concentrations of 12.9 ± 2.4 mg/L, 13.2 ± 2.7 mg/L and 13.2 ± 2.5 mg/L, respectively.

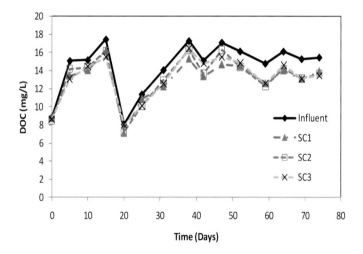

Figure 4.3 DOC concentrations of influent and effluent of soil columns during acclimation period (Influent: DCW+SE, HLR=0.64 m/d, column depth = 0.3 m, media size 0.8 – 1.25 mm, oxic conditions)

82

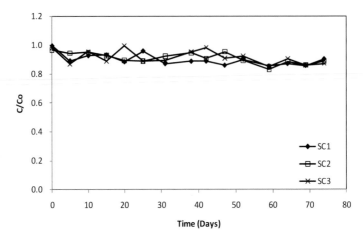

Figure 4.4 DOC removal in soil columns during acclimation period (Influent: DCW+SE, HLR=0.64 m/d, column depth= 0.3 m, media size 0.8 – 1.25 mm, oxic conditions).

4.3.3. SPE-Fluorescence detection of E2 and EE2

Estrogen compounds are generally determined by LC-MS/MS. However, LC-MS/MS method is expensive, time consuming and requires a high degree of analytical expertise. In this study, solid phase extraction (SPE, C18) followed by fluorescence was used to monitor E2 and EE2 at μg/L levels. SPE-fluorescence is not an accurate way to measure estrogen compounds at low levels in a natural sample. However, it can be used to monitor the fate of estrogen standards spiked in a water sample and can characterize dissolved organic matter (DOM) at the same time. Previously, fluorescence has been used to detect E2 and EE2 using high-performance liquid chromatography (HPLC) (excitation wavelength (Ex): 280 nm and emission wavelength (Em): 310 nm) (Yoon et al., 2003). Figure 4.5 shows the F-EEM of E2 (a) and EE2 (b) in Milli-Q-water. However, it is not possible to differentiate between estrogen compounds (e.g., E2 and EE2 or E1) using SPE-fluorescence.

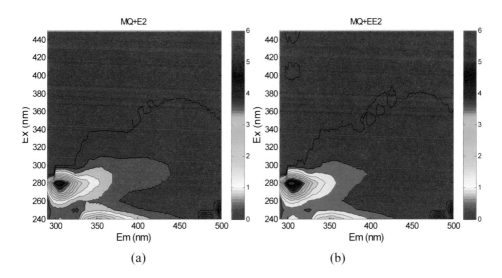

Figure 4.5 F-EEM spectra of (a) E2 and (b) EE2 standards with Milli-Q-water water (concentration = 1 mg/L)

E2

A calibration curve of E2 between 5 and 100 µg/L were prepared y using fluorescence (Ex: 280 nm and Em: 310 nm). The calibration curve of of E2 in Milli-Q-water showed R^2 of 0.95. Thus, E2 clearly showed a good correlation with fluorescence intensity, and fluorescence could be used to monitor the fate of E2. A mixture of DCW and SE (1:1) sample spiked with E2 standard at 100 µg/L of E2 was measured using SPE-fluorescence, and the sample without E2 standard (background) was also measured in a same way. The fluorescence spectra from the background sample was subtracted from the spiked sample, and the recovery of E2 was found to be 94 %. SPE (C18) improved the accuracy of E2 by eliminated organic matter that interferes with fluorescence intensity for E2. However, further study is needed to distinguish other estrogen compounds that may have similar fluorophore characteristics as E2 when the SPE-fluorescence method is used for unknown E2 samples. Therefore, the SPE-fluorescence method for estrogen compounds is limited to samples with a known estrogen. Figure 4.6 shows the fluorescence intensity observed from samples spiked with different E2 concentrations (50, 100, 150, 200 µg/L), and the intensity observed from recovery samples, correlated linearly with E2 concentration (R^2=0.97).

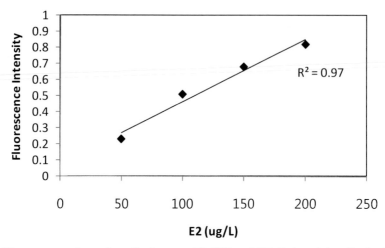

Figure 4.6 Fluorescence intensity of mixture of DCW and SE (1:1 ratio) spiked with E2 (50, 150, 100 and 200 µg/L)

EE2

The fluorescence peak at wavelengths of 280 nm (excitation) and 310 nm (emission) exhibited a good correlation to EE2 (R^2 = 0.99) (Figure 4.7). DCW and SE (1:1 ratio) samples spiked with different EE2 concentrations were also tested (50, 100, 150 and 200 µg/L). Thus, it is feasible to use SPE-fluorescence to investigate the fate of EE2 in a natural sample spiked with EE2 standard. Again, SPE-fluorescence cannot be applied to samples with unknown estrogens.

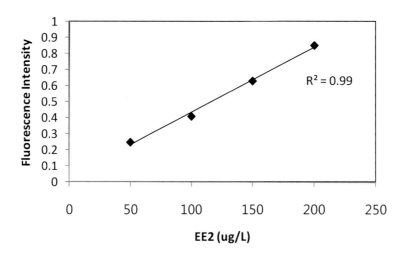

Figure 4.7 Fluorescence intensity of delft canal water and secondary effluent (1:1 ratio) spiked with EE2 (50, 100, 150 and 200 µg/L)

4.3.4. Abiotic batch experiment using sodium azide

Abiotic experiments using batch reactors were necessary to determine if it is feasible to use sodium azide as a biocide for abiotic conditions. Batch reactors were deployed as follows: 100 g of clean dry sand in eight batch reactors filled with secondary effluent up to 400 mL. 2 months of the acclimation period was necessary to stabilize batch reactors with respect to DOC removal (fill-and-draw mode during the acclimation period, HRT = 5 days). After the acclimation period, sodium azide at 2, 10 and 20 mM were added to batch reactors. DOC removals after 5-days is presented in Figure 4.8. ATP associated with sand indicated the microbial activity in the reactors, and DOC reduction did not significantly change in the control reactor (no sodium azide). However, the rest of reactors with sodium azide showed different behaviors of DOC. DOC did not change in the reactor with 2mM of sodium, but F-EEM indicated that there were increased protein-like peaks observed in samples fed with 10 and 20 mM of sodium azide (Figure 4.9b, 20 mM). According to Figure 4.9, protein-like substances increased under abiotic conditions. Batch reactors fed with 20 mM of sodium azide exhibited the lowest ATP concentration associated with sand. Thus, a sodium azide concentration of 20 mM was necessary to depress microbial activity associated with sand.

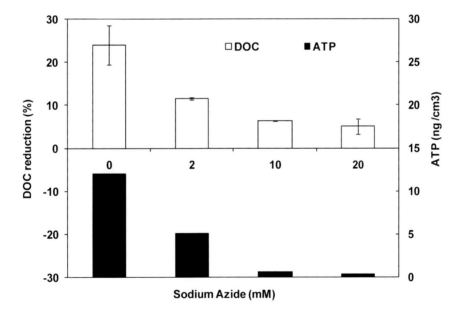

Figure 4.8 DOC removal in batch reactors with different concentration of the sodium azide: (HRT = 5 days)

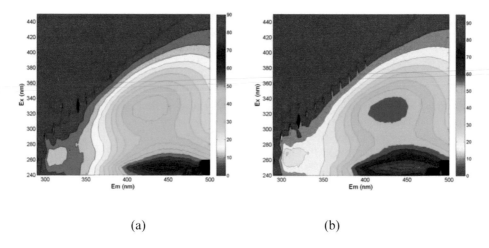

(a)   (b)

Figure 4.9 F-EEM spectra of samples from batch reactors under (a) biotic and (b) abiotic conditions using sodium azide (20 mM and HRT = 5 days)

4.3.5. Adsorption isotherms of E2 and EE2

Adsorption isotherms for E2 and EE2 were determined using Freundlich model. At the start, E2 and EE2 standards were added to influent (DCW and SE, 1:1) in the batch reactors with 100 g of silica sand (dry weight) in order to obtain initial E2 and EE2 concentrations of 20, 40, 80 and 100 μg/L. Batch reactors for E2 and EE2 were separately prepared due to interferences in ELISA analyses. Intermittent sampling for F-EEM allowed examining the behavior of E2 and EE2 over 5 days (HRT). All the reactors were maintained under oxic conditions. The adsorption capacity of sand (k) was 0.20 μg/g and adsorption intensity of sand (1/n) was 0.92 for E2 (Table 4.5). The 1/n is close to 1 which corresponds to a linear isotherm. The sorption of E2 by sand increased linearly with increasing concentration of E2 added to the reactors. The same experiment was conducted under biotic conditions for E2, and adsorption capacity of sand (k) and adsorption intensity of sand (1/n) were 2.88 μg/g and 0.57, respectively. Under biotic conditions, biomass associated with sand enhanced the adsorption of E2. For EE2, the adsorption capacity of sand (k) was 0.21 μg/g, and adsorption intensity of sand (1/n) was 0.63. log K_{ow} values of E2 and EE2 were 3.43 and 4.15, respectively. A high value of EE2 the more likely it will adsorb to soil particles. Under biotic conditions, the adsorption capacity of sand (k) was 0.22 μg/g, and the adsorption intensity of sand (1/n) was 0.68 for EE2.

Table 4.5 Freundlich isotherm parameters for adsorption of E2 and EE2 in secondary effluent onto acclimated sand under different conditions

Isotherm Parameters	E2		EE2	
	Oxic-abiotic	Oxic-biotic	Oxic-abiotic	Oxic-biotic
k (μg/g)	0.20	2.88	0.21	0.22
1/n	0.92	0.57	0.63	0.68

4.3.6. Factors affecting on the removal of E2 and EE2

Batch reactors were deployed to investigate factors that influence on the removal of E2 and EE2 during BF. Table 4.3 shows the summary of these experiments. Adsorption and biodegradation are the main removal mechanisms for E2 and EE2, but there are other factors that can influence the removal mechanisms of E2 and EE2. These factors are: 1) microbial activity and 2) redox conditions. As mentioned previously, the microbial activity associated with sand was determined by ATP. According to the abiotic experiment, sodium azide significantly decreased the microbial activity. Fresh sand (less biofilm) and tap water (very low carbon source) were also used to determine the role of microbial activity in the removal of E2 and EE2. Tap water in the Netherlands is biostable with assimilable organic carbon (AOC) of about 10 ug/L. E2 removal was not significantly different between biotic and abiotic conditions (Figure 4.10). It appears that adsorption was the main mechanism for E2 and EE2 due to their hydrophobicity (high K_{ow}). Moreover, redox conditions did not influence the removal of E2 as well (Figure 4.11). In a previous study, E2 and EE2 were degraded by microorganisms in aquifer material-water mixtures under aerobic and anoxic conditions (Ying et al., 2003). In our study, estrogenic activity remaining in a water sample under oxic conditions (13 ng EEQ/L) was relatively lower than that of under anoxic conditions (97 ng EEQ/L). Under oxic conditions, estrogenic activity was eliminated more rapidly compared with that of anoxic conditions.

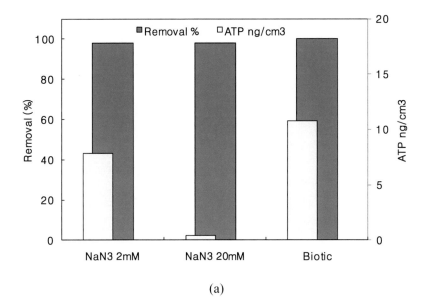

(a)

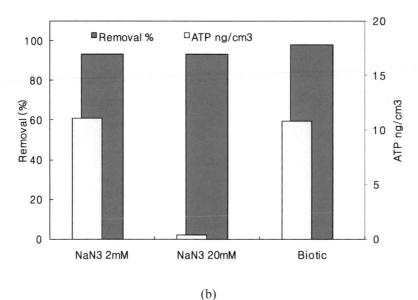

(b)

Figure 4.10 E2 (a) and EE2 (b) removal in batch reactors with acclimated sand under biotic and abiotic conditions (HRT = 5 days)

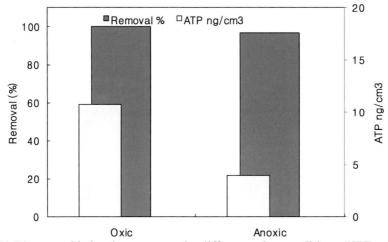

Figure 4.11 E2 removal in batch reactors under different redox conditions (HRT = 5 days)

Again, F-EEM detection at Ex 280 nm and Em 310 nm was used to determine the relative concentration of E2 at μg/L levels, and intermittent samples were taken from reactors. Figure 4.12 shows the fate of E2 in different reactors (a) Milli-Q water only, (b) effluent + acclimated sand and (c) effluent only without acclimated sand, and no significant change in estrogen peaks was found in the Milli-Q water. In case of the acclimated sand, the E2 peak was gradually reduced as time elapsed.

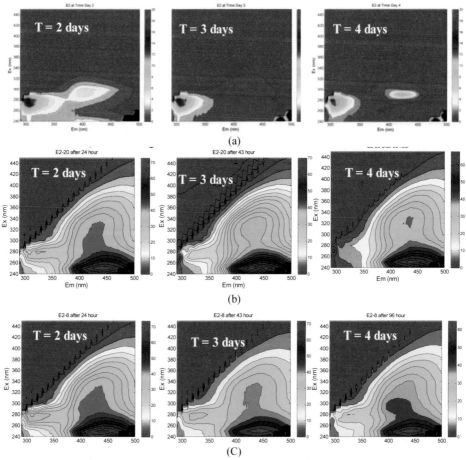

Figure 4.12 Fate of E2 during the batch experiment and effects of different conditions: (a) Milli-Q-water only, (b) DCW+SE with acclimated sand and (c) DCW+SE only

4.3.7. Soil column studies

Soil column studies were carried out to assess the fate of EE2 during soil passage. Three columns (SC1, SC2 and SC3) were deployed and the experiments were carried out in a dark room. The soil columns were 300 mm long comprised of inner and outer diameters (50 mm inner diameter, XK50/30, Amersham Pharmacia Biotech, Sweden). Silica sand (size 0.8 to 1.25 mm diameter) used as filter media and was acclimated for 60 days. The hydraulic loading rate was maintained at 0.64 m/day. SC-1 was fed with tap water (low carbon source), and DCW and SE (1:1) were introduced into SC2 and SC3. SC2 was maintained under abiotic conditions using sodium azide, and SC3 remained under biotic conditions. EE2 standard was spiked to maintain a concentration of 1 mg/L in the influent to SC1, SC2 and SC3, and samples were analyzed for EE2 concentrations using an ELISA kit. EE2 removals for SC1, SC2 and SC3 were 64%, 67% and 87%, respectively. SC1 was fed with tap water containing low organic matter (10 ug/L of AOC) under biotic conditions, and SC2 consisted of acclimated sand under abiotic conditions. It can be argued that the removals in SC1 and SC2 are mainly due to adsorption, and the removal in SC3 is due to the combination of adsorption and biodegradation. Adsorption appeared to be the major removal mechanism for EE2 removal, however the difference between SC2 and SC3 indicated that biodegradation also contributed to the reduction of EE2. In a previous study, EE2 was found to be degraded in an aquifer material acclimated with effluent (Ying et al., 2008). Therefore, adsorption and biodegradation are the main removal mechanisms that need to be considered when estimating the fate of EE2 during BF. It is hypothesized that EDCs first adsorb onto media and then slowly undergo biodegradation with time. Therefore, the adsorption capacity may be regenerated and not exhausted with time. Moreover, the EE2 removal was between 64 and 87% a depth of only 300 mm but higher removal is expected in BF system where travel distances are often greater than 10 m.

Table 4.6 Summary of soil column experiments (EBCT: 11 hours)

	SC1	SC2	SC3
Feed water	Non chlorinated tap water	DCW + SE (1:1 ratio)	DCW + SE (1:1 ratio)
Acclimation period (days)	60	60	60
Microbial activity	Biotic	Abiotic	Biotic
EE2 removal (%)	64	67	87

4.4. Conclusions

Based on the experimental results, the following conclusions can be drawn:

- Abiotic experiment using sodium azide depressed the microbial activity associated with sand. However, it is important to note that an abiotic experiment for BF needs careful consideration in inactivating microorganisms encapsulated in soil organic matter. Therefore, it is necessary to measure the microbial activity associated with the soil organic matter.

- The fluorescence peak which appeared at an excitation wavelength of 280 nm and emission wavelength of 310 nm detected E2 and EE2 in the range of μg/L.

- Pretreatment of a sample using solid phase extraction (SPE) is necessary to remove the bulk organic matter that interfered with E2 and EE2 fluorescence measurements. It was found that SPE-fluorescence can be used as a rapid method to monitor the fate of E2 and EE2.

- Batch experiments showed a significant removal of E2, E1 and EE2, and estrogenic activity measured by ER-CALUX indicated that most of the remaining estrogenic activity (ng estradiol-equivalents (EEQ)/L) in filtrates was eliminated.

- Redox conditions did not influence the removal of E2 and EE2. However, estrogenic activity remaining in a filtrate under oxic conditions (13 ng EEQ /L) was relatively lower than that under anoxic conditions (97 ng EEQ /L).

- Soil column studies showed that EE2 removals for SC1, SC2 and SC3 were 64%, 67% and 87%, respectively. Adsorption appeared to be the major removal mechanism for EE2. However, the difference of EE2 removal between SC2 (abiotic) and SC3 (biotic) revealed that biodegradation also contributed to the reduction of EE2.

- BF is an effective way to attenuate E2, E1 and EE2. Estrogen compounds selected in this study are hydrophobic compounds and biodegradable compounds; thus, a treatment process such as BF, based on adsorption and biodegradation, is effective.

4.5. References

Andersen H., Siegrist H., Halling-sørensen B. and Ternes T., 2003. Fate of Estrogens in a municipal sewage treatment plant. Environ. Sci. Technol. 37, 4021.

Birkett. J.W., 2003. Sources of endocrine disrupter IWS Publishing & Lewis Publishers, London.

Blaber S.J.M., 1970. The occurrence of a penis-like outgrowth behind the right tentacle in spent females of Nucella lapillus. Proc. Malac. Soc. London 39, 231-233.

Carballa M., Omil F., Lema J.M., Llompart M., García-Jares C., Rodríguez I., Gómez M. and Ternes T., 2004. Behavior of pharmaceuticals, cosmetics and hormones in a sewage treatment plant. Water Res. 38, 2918-2926.

Cargouët M., Peridiz D., Mouatassim-Souali A., Tamisier-Karolak S. and Levi Y., 2004 Assessment of river contamination by estrogenic compounds in Paris area (France). Sci. Total Environ. 324, 55-66.

Colborn T. and Clement C., 1992. Chemically induced alteration in sexual development: the wildlife/human connection. Princeton Scientific Publishing Company, Princeton NJ.

Czajka C.P. and Londry K.L., 2006. Anaerobic biotransformation of estrogens. Sci. Total Environ., 367(2-3), 932-941.

Gomes R.L. and Lester J.N., 2003. Endocrine Disrupters in Receiving Waters IWA Publishing & Lewis Publishers, London.

Hanselman T.A., Graetz D.A. and Wilkie A.C., 2003. Manure-Borne estrogens as potential environmental contaiminants: A review. Environ. Sci. Technol. 37, 5471-5478.

Hintemann T., Schneider C., Schöler H. and Schneider R., 2006. Field study using two immunoasays for the determination of estadiol and ethinylestradiol in the aquatic environment. Water Res. 40, 2287-2294.

Khanal S.K., Xie B., Thompson M.L., Sung S., Ong S.-K. and Leeuwen J.V., 2006. Fate, and transport and biodegradation of natural estrogens in the environment and engineerin systems. Environ. Sci. Technol. 40, 6537-6545.

Layton A.C., Gregory B.W., Seward J.R., Schultz T.W. and Sayler G.S., 2000. Mineralization of steridal hormones by biosolids in wastewater treatment system in Tennesse U.S.A. Environ. Sci. Technol. 34, 3925-3931.

Legler J., Dennekamp M., Vethaak A.D., Brouwer A., Koeman J.H., van der Burg B. and Murk A.J., 2002. Detection of estrogenic activity in sediment-associated compounds using in vitro reporter gene assays. Sci. Total Environ. 293, 69-83.

Lishman L., Smyth S.A., Sarafin K., Kleywegt S., Toito J., Peart T., Lee B., Servos M., Beland M. and Seto P., 2006. Occurrence and reductions of pharmaceuticals and personal care products and estrogens by municipal wastewater treatment plants in Ontario, Canada. Sci. Total Environ. 367(2-3), 544-558.

Ma, M., Rao, K. and Wang, Z., 2007. Occurrence of estrogenic effects in sewage and industrial wastewaters in Beijing, China. Environ. Pollut. 147(2), 331-336.

Mansell J., Drewes J.E. and Rauch T., 2004. Removal mechanism of endocrine disrupting compounds (steriods) soil aquifer treatment. Water Sci. Technol. 50, 229.

Nakada N., Yasojima M., Miyajima K., Komori K., Suzuki Y. and Tanaka H., 2005. Fate of estrogenic compounds and estrogenic activity in wastewater treatment process, Technology 2005 2nd Joint Specialty Conference for Sustainable Management of Water Quality Systems for the 21st Century: Working to Project Public Health, Water Environment Federation, San Francisco, USA.

Sarmah A.K., Northcott G.L., Leusch F.D.L. and Tremblay L.A., 2006. A study of endocrine disrupting cheicals (EDCs) in municipal sewage and amimal waste effluents in the Waikato region of New Zealand. Sci. Total Environ. 355, 135-144.

Shappel N.W., 2006. Estrogenic activity in the environment: muniicipal wastewater effluent, river, ponds and wetlands. J. Environ. Qual. 35, 122-132.

Smith B.S., 1971. Sexuality in the american mud snail, Nassarius obsoletus. Proc. Malac. Soc. London 39, 377-378.

Suzuki Y. and Maruyama T., 2006. Fate of natural estrogens in bathc mixing experiment using municipal sewage and activated sludge. Water Res. 40, 1061-1069.

Ternes T.A., Stumpf M., Mueller J., Haberer K. and Wilken R.-D., 1999. Behavior and occurence of estrogens in municipal sewage treatment plant - I. Investigations in Germany, Canada and Brazil. Sci. Total Environ. 225, 81-90.

Ying G.-G., Kookana R.S. and Dillon P., 2003. Sorption and degradation of selected five endocrine disrupting chemicals in aquifer material. Water Res. 37, 3785-3791.

Ying G.-G., Toze S., Hanna J., Yu X.-Y., Dillon P.J. and Kookana R.S. 2008. Decay of endocrine-disrupting chemicals in aerobic and anoxic groundwater. Water Res. 42, 1133-1141.

Yoon Y., Westerhoff P., Snyder S.A. and Esparza M., 2003. HPLC-fluorescence detection and adsorption of bisphenol A, 17[beta]-estradiol, and 17[alpha]-ethynyl estradiol on powdered activated carbon. Water Res. 37, 3530-3537.

Chapter 5

ROLE OF BIODEGRADATION IN THE REMOVAL OF PHARMACEUTICALLY ACTIVE COMPOUNDS DURING BANK FILTRATION

Parts of this chapter are based on:

Yangali-Quintanilla, V., Maeng, S.K., Fujioka, T., Kennedy, M., Amy, G.L., 2010. Proposing nanofiltration as acceptable barrier for organic contaminants in water reuse, Journal of Membrane Science, 362, 334-345.

Sharma, S.K., Maeng, S.K., Nam, S., Amy, G.L., 2011. Chapter 68. Characterization Tools for Differentiating NOM from EfOM. In "Treatise on Water Science", Volume 3: Aquatic Chemistry and Microbiology, Elsevier Publications (In Press)

Summary

Natural treatment systems such bank filtration have been recognized as an effective barrier in the multi-barrier approach for the attenuation of organic micropollutants for safe drinking water supply. In this study, the role of biodegradation in removing selected pharmaceutically active compounds (PhACs) during soil passage was investigated. Firstly, batch studies were conducted to investigate the removal of 13 selected PhACs from different water sources with respect to different sources of biodegradable organic matter. Column experiments were then performed to differentiate between biodegradation and sorption in the removal of selected PhACs. Selected neutral PhACs (phenacetine, paracetamol and caffeine) and acidic PhACs (ibuprofen, fenoprofen, bezafibrate and naproxen) exhibited removal efficiencies of greater than 87% from different organic matter water matrices during batch studies (contact time: 60 days). In column studies, removal efficiencies of acidic PhACs (e.g., analgesics) decreased under biodegradable carbon-limited conditions. Removal efficiencies of selected acidic PhACs (ibuprofen, fenoprofen, bezafibrate, ketoprofen and naproxen) were less than 35% under abiotic conditions. These removals were attributed to sorption under abiotic conditions established by a biocide (20 mM sodium azide), which suppressed microbial activity/biodegradation. However, under biotic conditions, removal efficiencies of these acidic PhACs compounds were greater than 78%, mainly attributed to biodegradation. Moreover, average removal efficiencies of hydrophilic (polar) neutral PhACs with low octanol/water partition coefficients (log K_{ow} less than 2) (paracetamol, pentoxifylline, phenacetine and caffeine) were low (< 12 %) under abiotic conditions. However, under biotic conditions, removal efficiencies of the neutral PhACs were greater than 91%. In contrast, carbamazepine showed a persistent behavior under both biotic and abiotic conditions. Overall, this study found that biodegradation was an important mechanism for the removal of PhACs during soil passage.

5.1. Introduction

During recent years, there has been a growing concern over the increased detection of organic micropollutants (OMPs) including pharmaceutically active compounds (PhACs), endocrine disrupting compounds (EDCs), and personal care products (PCPs) in drinking water and the aquatic environment. The growing use of PhACs, EDCs and PCPs for human and veterinary purposes has increased the frequency of detection in water supplies and the environment (Heberer, 2002; Jjemba, 2006). Currently, the total consumption of PhACs, EDCs and PCPs in the world is not known because many of these compounds significantly vary with respect to application and consumption from one country to another (Cunningham, 2004). Also, the development of new analytical procedures and instruments enables analysts to quantify the level of environmental contamination to much lower concentrations, contributing to an increased number of detections of OMPs in the aquatic environment and drinking water (Snyder et al., 2004). Generally, PhACs, EDCs and PCPs remain as a mixture in the environment; thus, these compounds might have different, possibly synergistic, impacts on public health and/or aquatic life compared to when a single compound exists (Kümmerer, 2009).

Major routes of PhACs and metabolites, which are formed as by-products during ingestion (i.e., biochemical reactions), into the environment are excretion in association with both urine and feces. Non-point sources such as overland flow (i.e., runoff) by heavy rainfall or land drainage in agriculture can also deliver PhACs (e.g., veterinary medicines) to surface waters or ground waters (Boxall et al., 2004). However, little is known about the fate of PhACs and metabolites (i.e., by-products) during drinking water treatment processes and in the aquatic environment (Mompelat et al., 2009). This, therefore, creates the possibility of the occurrence of potentially harmful pollutants such as EDCs in drinking water sources.

The occurrence of PhACs in drinking water sources has resulted in increased research on PhACs and the use of advanced technologies to provide a reliable supply of safe drinking water (Kim et al., 2007; Madden et al., 2009; Mechlinski and Heberer, 2005; Mompelat et al., 2009; Yangali-Quintanilla et al., 2010). The removal of PhACs from water is relatively costly with advanced water treatment technologies, thus leading to a high unit cost of water treatment. However, managed aquifer recharge (MAR) treatment processes such as riverbank filtration (RBF), lake bank filtration (LBF) and artificial recharge (AR) are robust and cost-effective treatments for some degree of OMP removal. Previous field studies have shown that RBF, LBF and AR are effective for OMP removal (Grünheid and Jekel, 2005; Heberer et al., 2004; Massmann et al., 2008; Mechlinski and Heberer, 2005; Schmidt et al., 2007).

There are a number of mechanisms which drive PhACs removal during soil passage. The most important mechanism in the elimination of PhACs is biodegradation. Moreover, biodegradability of PhACs is an important aspect of assessing their fate and risk under environmental conditions (Cunningham, 2004). The biodegradation of PhACs is the most desirable removal mechanism because it is a sustainable process and potentially results in end-products consisting of inorganic compounds (i.e., mineralization) (Howard, 2000). Another important mechanism of PhACs removal during RBF is sorption, which impacts the bioavailability of PhACs. The octanol/water partition coefficient (K_{ow}) is often used to assess the sorption potential and distribution behavior of OMPs in the aquatic environment. However, K_{ow} may not properly describe the distribution behavior between soil and water for some acidic PhACs (i.e., electrostatic interactions). Many non-steroidal anti-inflammatory drugs (NSAIDs) and lipid regulators are acidic PhACs and remain in ionized forms at environmentally relevant pH levels (Cunningham, 2004). Therefore, the acid dissociation constant (pK_a) of acidic PhACs and the pH of the aquatic environment are important to understand the fate of acidic PhACs during soil passage.

Many previous studies have attempted to examine the removal of PhACs by sorption, photolysis and biodegradation in wastewater, secondary effluent or surface water. However, there has been little research to investigate the effect of the biodegradable fraction of natural organic matter (NOM) on PhACs removal using a suite of innovative NOM analytical tools (e.g., fluorescence excitation-emission matrices (F-EEM), liquid chromatography with an on-line organic carbon detection (LC-OCD), etc.) as well as comparison between sorption and biodegradation of PhACs during soil passage. The objective of this study was to investigate the role of biodegradation in the removal of 13 selected PhACs during soil passage. Additionally, the removal of different classes of PhACs from different water matrices (i.e., different NOM characteristics) was examined.

5.2. Materials and methods

5.2.1. Chemicals

Thirteen (13) selected PhACs (gemfibrozil, diclofenac, bezafibrate, ibuprofen, fenoprofen, naproxen, ketoprofen, clofibric acid, carbamazepine, phenacetine, paracetamol, pentoxifylline and caffeine) were used to prepare stock solutions, out of which working solutions were made and spiked into different experimental setups. Using Milli-Q water (Advantage A10, Millipore), stock solutions of 100 µg/L concentration were prepared. All PhACs under investigation were of analytical grade and purchased from Sigma–Aldrich, Germany. Physicochemical properties of selected compounds are shown in Table 5.1. For acidic pharmaceuticals, log D was used an indicator of their hydrophobicity. According to Cunningham (2004), a chemical with log D values less than 1 is unlikely sorb onto organic matter or bioconcentrate (hydrophilic), whereas a chemical with log D equal or higher than 1 may significantly bioconcentrate or sorb onto/into soil organic matter (hydrophobic). For neutral pharmaceuticals, log K_{ow} was used in the same way as log D. Easily biodegradable synthetic organic matter (SOM) was used as an external carbon sources for a batch experiment. It was prepared from aldehydes (formaldehyde 200 µg/L and glyoxal 60 µg/L) and carboxylic acids (sodium acetate 800 µg/L and sodium formate 600 µg/L) and then used for column studies. The composition of the SOM was based on the formation of organic by-products from ozonation (Urfer and Huck, 2001). However, the concentrations of organic by-products used in this study were higher than the concentrations originating from a full-scale drinking water plant using ozonation (Urfer and Huck, 2001).

Table 5.1 List of PhACs studied and their properties

Name	MW (g/mol)	pK_a	log K_{ow}[1]	log D[2] (pH=8)	Classification @ pH=8[3]
Gemfibrozil	250.3	4.7	4.77	2.22	Hydrophobic-Ionic
Diclofenac	296.2	4.2	4.51	1.59	Hydrophobic-Ionic
Bezafibrate	361.8	3.6	4.25	0.69	Hydrophilic-Ionic
Ibuprofen	206.3	4.9	3.97	1.44	Hydrophobic-Ionic
Fenoprofen	242.3	4.5	3.9	1.11	Hydrophobic-Ionic
Naproxen	230.3	4.2	3.18	0.05	Hydrophilic-Ionic
Ketoprofen	254.3	4.5	3.12	0.41	Hydrophilic-Ionic
Clofibric acid	214.6	3.2	2.88	-1.08	Hydrophilic-Ionic
Carbamazepine	236.3	n.a.	2.45	-	Hydrophilic-Neutral
Phenacetine	179.2	n.a.	1.67	-	Hydrophilic-Neutral
Paracetamol	151.2	n.a.	0.27	-	Hydrophilic-Neutral
Pentoxifylline	278.3	n.a.	0.29	-	Hydrophilic-Neutral
Caffeine	194.2	n.a.	-0.07	-	Hydrophilic-Neutral

[1] KOWWIN v.1.67 (US EPA, 2009)
[2] ADME/Tox WEB software (http://www.pharma-algorithms.com/webboxes/)
[3] For acidic pharmaceuticals: hydrophobic: log D > 1, hydrophilic: log D < 1 at pH 8; for neutral pharmaceuticals: hydrophobic: log K_{ow} > 2, hydrophilic: K_{ow} < 2

5.2.2. Batch experimental setups

Batch experiments (1 liter glass bottles) using silica sand (grain size 0.8 - 1.25 mm) were used to assess attenuation of selected PhACs using different sources of water, simulating long residence time (e.g., 60 days consisted of oxic (30 days) followed by anoxic (30 days) conditions) during RBF. Five batch reactors in triplicate were used together with five different water types: (1) the river Meuse water, The Netherlands (MR), (2) the river Meuse water spiked with synthetic organic matter (SOM) as an additional carbon sources (MR+SOM), (3) secondary effluent from wastewater treatment plant, Hoek van Holland, The Netherlands (SE), (4) water from an experimental container used for cultivation of the common reed, *Phragmites australis* (CR), (5) non-chlorinated tap water (NCTW), Delft, The Netherlands (assimilable organic carbon close to 10 ug/L). For the CR, *Phragmites australis* was excavated from the shore of a lake located in Delft, The Netherlands and (trans) planted in a specially-constructed container. The water level of the container was maintained at the container surface. The plants were incubated under constant temperature (16∘C) with a 14-hr light period. CR was collected from the valve located at the bottom of the container. The intent of using CR for batch reactors was to simulate water with high contents of humic substances. CR exhibited high aromaticity from SUVA analysis and CR contained organic matter which originated from soil organic matter.

Initially, batch reactors fed with MR, MR+SOM, SE or CR were bioacclimated with their respective influents until the reactors stabilized (i.e., acclimated) with respect to dissolved organic carbon (DOC) reduction. Then, each reactor was spiked with selected PhACs in concentrations ranging from 1.8 µg/L and 5.4 µg/L. All batch reactors were placed on a shaker table and rotated at 100 rpm under oxic conditions (30 days) followed by anoxic conditions (30 days) (i.e., total residence times of 60 days). Generally, redox conditions during RBF exhibit oxic conditions followed by anoxic conditions along the flow transect. Therefore, after the first 30 days under oxic conditions, nitrogen gas was used to remove dissolved oxygen (DO) from batch reactors using sparger diffusers which were designed for a HPLC system (i.e., DO < 0.2 mg/L). Nitrogen gas was very gently introduced to prevent any disturbance in batch reactors. After 60 days, nitrate concentrations were still remained in the reactors that there was no other electron acceptors used beyond nitrate. A blank experiment was also performed by taking approximately the same concentration of PhACs used for batch reactors in Milli-Q water without silica sand in order to investigate the degree of PhACs loss (i.e., sorption on the glassware). The average loss of PhACs during the control experiment was determined to be less than 7%.

5.2.3. Column experimental setups

Double-walled soil columns (SC) (XK50/30, Amersham Pharmacia Biotech, Sweden) of 50 mm inner diameter and 300 mm length were used. The inner part of the columns was packed with silica sand (0.8 – 1.25 mm), while the outer part was used to control the ambient temperature by flowing water from a chiller. All SCs were kept in a dark room to minimize potential effects of photodegradation. Four sand columns (SC1, SC2, SC3 and SC4) were deployed to assess the role of biodegradation in the removal of PhACs and compared with sorption. All four columns were connected to a chiller, whereby operating temperatures were maintained between 16°C to 17°C. Empty bed contact time (EBCT) for the SC set-up was 11 hours which was determined by tracer study using NaCl (hydraulic loading rate: 0.64 m/day). Before introducing selected PhACs, SC1 and SC2 were bioacclimated with MR for two months. Like in case of batch experiment mentioned above, the acclimation process was continued until both columns stabilized with respect to DOC reduction. After the acclimation period, NCTW and MR with PhACs served as the feed to the SC1 and the SC2, respectively. The SC1 aimed at assessment of biodegradation of selected PhACs under low microbial conditions using NCTW (i.e., low biodegradable organic matter). If some selected PhACs are removed by co-metabolism, carbon limited conditions may diminish their removal efficiencies in SC1. In contrast to the acclimation period of 60 days for SC1 and SC2 , SC3 had only 10 days to have less active biomass associated with sand. SC4 was packed with fresh sand, fed with demineralized water (DW) containing sodium azide (NaN$_3$, 20 mM) to maintain the column under abiotic conditions, and it was used to investigate the removal of PhACs by sorption. Sodium azide was used to suppress microbial activity in SC4. Adenosine triphosphate (ATP) and DOC concentrations were measured to verify that the SC4 column was maintained under abiotic conditions.

Sodium azide is a biocide frequently used to suppress microbial activity for abiotic experiments (i.e., sorption experiments) (Chen et al., 2008; Liang et al., 2006).

5.2.4. Analytical methodology

Dissolved organic matter (DOM) in all samples was characterized within 3 days after samples were collected and stored under 5°C after 0.45 µm filtration (Whatman, Dassel, Germany) to prevent biodegradation of DOM. The concentration of DOM was determined as DOC by a total organic carbon analyzer (Shimadzu TOC-V$_{CPN}$). The characteristics of DOM were elucidated by various analytical methods including fluorescence excitation-emission matrix (F-EEM), liquid chromatography with an on-line organic carbon detection (LC-OCD) (DOC-LABOR Dr. Huber, Karlsruhe, Germany) and specific ultraviolet absorbance (SUVA). In F-EEM, all samples were adjusted to 1 mg/L of DOC by diluting samples with Milli-Q water and measured by a FluoroMax-3 spectrofluorometer (HORIBA Jobin Yvon, Edison, NJ, USA). F-EEM spectra were obtained at excitation wavelengths between 240 nm to 450 nm in 10-nm intervals and emission wavelengths between 290 nm and 500 nm in 2-nm intervals. Also, the water Raman peak at 348 nm was used to confirm the stability of the spectrofluorometer, and F-EEM were corrected using blank subtraction. Table 5.2 and Figure 5.1 show the characteristics of DOM expressed as regions determined by distinct wavelengths of excitation and emission (Coble, 1996; Henderson et al., 2009; Leenheer and Croue, 2003). A LC-OCD system uses a liquid chromatography method describing the molecular weight (MW) distribution and classification of DOM according to biopolymers, humic substances, building blocks, low MW acids, and neutrals. More details of this system have been described in Huber and Frimmel (1992). UV absorbance was measured at 254 nm by a UV/Vis spectrophotometer (UV-2501PC Shimadzu), and SUVA was calculated by dividing UV$_{254}$ absorbance by DOC concentration to represent the relative aromaticity of organic matter.

Table 5.2 Characteristics of organic matter using 3 key fluorescence peaks (primary humic-like peak (P1), secondary humic-like peak (P2) and protein-like peak (P3)) in F-EEM

	Excitation (nm)	Emission (nm)	Description	References
P1	250-260	380-480	Humic-like substances (Primary)	(Leenheer and Croue 2003)
	237-260	400-500		(Coble 1996)
P2	330-350	420-480	Humic-like substances (Secondary)	(Leenheer and Croue 2003)
	300-370	400-500		(Coble 1996)
P3	270-280	320-350	Tryptophan-like, Protein-like substances	(Leenheer and Croue 2003)
	275	340		(Coble 1996)
	280	350		(Henderson et al. 2009)

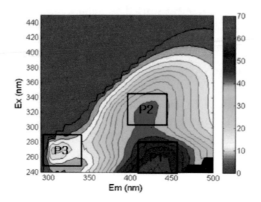

Figure 5.1 Typical F-EEM spectra of secondary effluent with three characteristic peaks

Adenosine triphosphate (ATP) was used to determine active microbial biomass (AMB) associated with sand in this study (Oades and Jenkinson, 1979). Wet sand samples of 1 to 2 g, collected from batch and column studies, were suspended in autoclaved tap water (50 mL). High energy sonication at a power of 40W was applied to detach the biomass (Branson W-250D Sonifier, microtip D ¼ 5 mm). The biomass concentration was determined as the concentration of ATP in the suspension obtained by the sonication. A single 2-minute sonication treatment was adequate to obtain more than 90% of the attached biomass represented as ATP (data not shown). A detailed description of methods and materials used for ATP extraction is explained in Magic-Knezev and van der Kooij (2004).

For PhAC measurements, autotrace SPE workstations from Caliper Life Sciences GmbH (Rüsselsheim, Germany) were used for solid phase extraction. HPLC-ESI-MS-MS measurements were performed on a HPLC system 1100, series II from Agilent Technologies (Waldbronn, Germany) equipped with an API 2000 triple quadrupole mass spectrometer from PE Sciex (Langen, Germany) using electrospray ionisation (ESI) under atmospheric pressure. The details of this analytical method are given elsewhere (Sacher et al., 2008).

5.3. Results and discussion

5.3.1. Removal of selected PhACs from different water sources: batch experiments

Dissolved organic matter characteristics

Five batch reactors in triplicate were used to investigate attenuation of PhACs using different water sources (e.g., MR, MR+SE (1:1), SE, NCTW and CR) spiked with

PhACs (total residence time 60 days: oxic (30 days) and anoxic conditions (30 days)). Samples were taken from each batch reactor at the beginning and at the end of the incubation period and were analyzed for pH, DOC, UV_{254} and SUVA. Table 5.3 shows organic matter characteristics of influents and effluents from batch studies. $BDOC_{60-day}$ was defined by the DOC change during 60 days of incubation. SE exhibited the highest $BDOC_{60-day}$ value of 6.3 ± 0.5 mg/L followed by CR (4.6 ± 1.9 mg/L), MR+SOM (2.8 ± 0.4 mg/L) and MR (1.5 ± 0.2 mg/L). $BDOC_{60-day}$ values for batch reactors were higher than $BDOC_{5-day}$ (contact time: 5 days) measured during the time of acclimation because of the slowly biodegradable organic matter which degrades over longer residence times.

Table 5.3 Characteristics of influent and effluent for batch reactors

		pH	DOC (mg/L)	$BDOC_{60-day}$ (mg/L)*	% BDOC to DOC	UV_{254} (ab./cm)	SUVA (L/mg-m)
NCTW	Influent	7.75	2.0	0.5	25		
	Effluent	7.98	1.5				
MR	Influent	7.73	3.6	1.5	42	0.11	3.12
	Effluent	8.33	2.1			0.09	4.26
MR+SOM	Influent	7.77	5.3	2.8	53	0.12	2.36
	Effluent	8.42	2.5			0.11	4.72
CR	Influent	7.87	14.6	4.6	32	0.53	3.61
	Effluent	8.48	10.0			0.39	3.94
SE	Influent	7.62	14.8	6.3	43	0.50	3.41
	Effluent	8.61	8.5			0.42	4.96

*DOC_{60-day} - DOC_{0-day}

SUVA values of 3.61 L/mg-m for CR followed by SE (3.41 L/mg-m) and MR (3.12 L/mg-m), indicates the aromaticity (humic content) of organic matter in each sample. The low SUVA value observed in MR+SOM (2.36 L/mg-m) was attributed to the aliphatic nature of SOM added to the MR. The residence time of 60 days in bioactive sand resulted in an increase of SUVA, due to the biodegradation of the aliphatic components of DOM in the samples. Previous studies have also shown similar results (Cha et al., 2004; Xue et al., 2009). Cha et al. (2004) showed that SUVA values increased in effluents from columns filled with natural river soil, due to biodegradation of aliphatic organic matter. The dominant fraction of organic matter in CR appeared to be the high content of humic substances which resulted in only a small increase in SUVA value during the 60 days of incubation time.

F-EEM spectra of influent and effluent samples were measured to probe the changes in characteristics of DOM during batch studies. Contour lines represent the distribution of fluorescence intensities at different excitation-emission wavelengths (Figure 5.1). As mentioned before, a F-EEM spectrum shows fluorescence intensity (FI) peaks at known wavelengths such that a FI peak at higher values of excitation (Ex) and emission (Em) wavelengths corresponds to humic-like substances, whereas an FI peak at lower values of Ex and Em wavelengths corresponds to protein-like substances (Amy and Drewes, 2007). Three peaks were identified: a primary humic-like peak, P1 (Ex/Em = 250-270/420-440 nm), a secondary humic-like peak, P2 (Ex/Em = 330-340/420-440 nm), and a protein-like peak, P3 (Ex/Em = 270-280/320-340 nm). Based on these peaks, the differences between FIs (ambient DOC) at time = 0 day and time = 60 days were calculated and compared to investigate the transformation of DOM. Results of F-EEM spectra of batch reactors are shown in Figure 5.2 through Figure 5.5. After 60 days of contact time, there were substantial decreases in P3 for MR, MR+SOM and SE. According to a previous study done by Hudson et al. (2008), the tryptophan-like peak (i.e., protein-like peak, EX/EM = 275/340 nm) was found to be an accurate surrogate for the presence and relative proportions of bioavailable organic matter. In this study, this tryptophan-like peak was found at EX/EM = 270-280/320-340 nm. In contrast, the FI of P1 and P2 increased for MR, MR+SOM and SE, except for CR.

Figure 5.2 exhibited an increase in P1 and P2 by 27% and 34%, respectively, whilst 52% of P3 was removed for MR. In addition, 36% of the DOC was removed from the MR. Figure 5.3 also showed increases in FI by 63% and 64% for humic-like peaks P1 and P2, respectively, for MR+SOM. On the other hand, the removal of the protein-like peak P3 was equal to that of the MR (52%), and DOC removal for the MR+SOM was found to be 44%. For SE, the FI for P1 and P2 increased by 32% and 25%, respectively, for SE (Figure 5.4). Again, the protein-like peak P3 was reduced by 49.3%, and DOC removal was 34%. Figure 5.5 indicates that relatively small increases of P1 (3%) and P2 (6%) were observed for CR. Moreover, DOC was removed by 18%, while P3 was removed by 48%. These results indicate that the FI values for P1 and P2 do not correlate to the reduction in DOC concentrations for 60 days of contact time. In fact, this result describes the biotransformation of DOM, and the degree of DOM biotransformation in CR was relatively small compared to MR, MR+SOM and SE.

According to Saadi et al. (2006), new fluorescing materials associated with DOM (i.e., fluorescing DOM) are formed in effluent-inoculated samples during long-term biodegradation (i.e., time = 60 days). They showed that certain organic components in DOM were able to biotransform into fluorescing DOM. Such increases in fluorescence were also observed in our study for P2 and P3 (i.e., humic-like substances) for MR, MR+SOM and SE samples during 60 days of contact time. According to our previous column studies, the FI of P2 and P3 did not increase during a short contact time (e.g., HRT = 5 days) (Maeng et al., 2008). Therefore, the formation of fluorescing DOM was minimal during the short contact time, and this fraction was small compared to the degradation of fluorescing DOM. However, during a long contact time (i.e., 60 days), slowly biodegradable compounds significantly contributed to the formation of fluorescing DOM to a greater level than the degradation of fluorescing DOM. Moreover, it was also found that formation of fluorescing DOM is not only limited by the contact time which allows slowly biodegradable organic matter to be degraded, but also the type of DOM which can be easily biotransformed into new fluorescing DOM. The F-EEM of the MR+SOM showed relatively high increases (63% and 64% for P1 and P2, respectively) for P1 and P2 compared to the other water types. This is attributed to

SOM (i.e., organic by-products from ozonation) that were easily biotransformed into new fluorescing DOM. Ogawa et al. (2001) found out that marine bacteria are able to form refractory DOM (i.e., fluorescing aromatic organic matter) from labile compounds (glucose and glumate). On the other hand, the formation of fluorescing DOM was not observed in CR samples, due to the aromatic nature of the organic matter (i.e., not readily biodegradable).

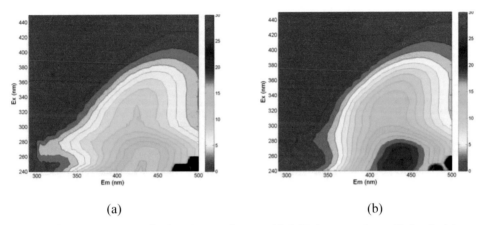

(a)   (b)

Figure 5.2 F-EEM spectra for batch experiment with MR (contact time: 60 days): (a) influent and (b) effluent

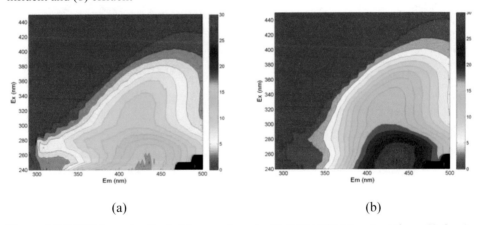

(a)   (b)

Figure 5.3 F-EEM spectra for batch experiment with MR+SOM (contact time: 60 days): (a) influent and (b) effluent

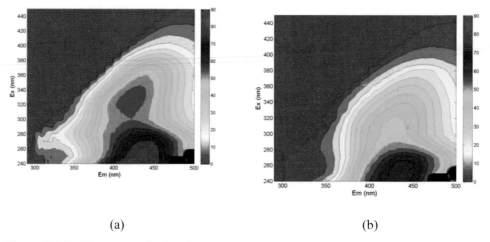

(a)   (b)

Figure 5.4 F-EEM spectra for batch experiment with SE (contact time: 60 days): (a) influent and (b)   effluent

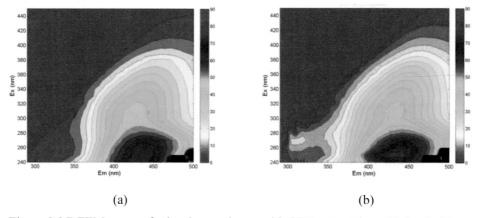

(a)   (b)

Figure 5.5 F-EEM spectra for batch experiment with CR (contact time: 60 days): (a) influent and (b) effluent

Differential spectra of FI (ambient DOC) between influent and effluent samples were calculated and shown in Figure 5.6 to Figure 5.9. Two types of differential spectra were calculated between influent and effluent samples. First, the spectrum of each effluent from MR, MR+SOM, SE and CR was subtracted from their influent spectrum to represent degradation of fluorescing NOM (Figure 5.6a, Figure 5.7a, Figure 5.8a and Figure 5.9a). Secondly, the spectrum of each influent from MR, MR+SOM, SE and CR was subtracted from their effluent spectrum to represent formation of fluorescing NOM (Figure 5.6b, Figure 5.7b, Figure 5.8b and Figure 5.9b). As shown from Figure 5.6 to Figure 5.9, the degradation of fluorescing DOM mainly occurred in P3 (i.e., protein-like substances), however, a significant increase of fluorescing DOM occurred in P1 and P2 during a long contact time.

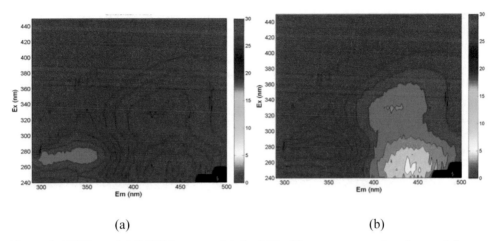

(a)   (b)

Figure 5.6 Differential F-EEM spectra (a) the MR effluent spectrum is subtracted from its influent spectrum to show degradation of fluorescing DOM, (b) the MR influent spectrum is subtracted from its effluent spectrum to show formation of fluorescing DOM

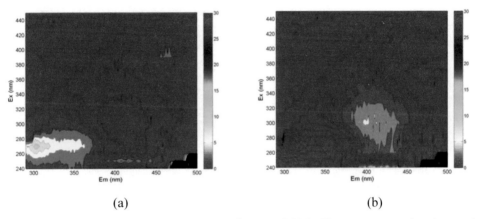

(a)   (b)

Figure 5.7 Differential F-EEM spectra (a) the MR+SOM effluent spectrum is subtracted from its influent spectrum to show degradation of fluorescing DOM, (b) the MR+SOM influent spectrum is subtracted from its effluent spectrum to show formation of fluorescing DOM

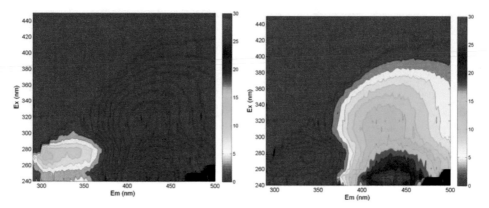

Figure 5.8 Differential F-EEM spectra (a) the SE effluent spectrum is subtracted from its influent spectrum to show degradation of fluorescing DOM, (b) the SE influent spectrum is subtracted from its effluent spectrum to show formation of fluorescing DOM

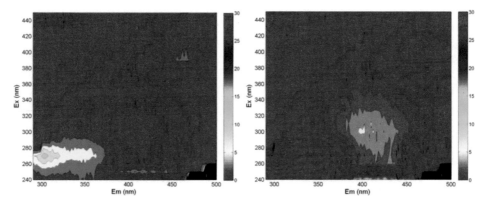

Figure 5.9 F-EEM spectra (a) the CR effluent spectrum is subtracted from its influent spectrum to show degradation of fluorescing DOM, (b) the CR influent spectrum is subtracted from its effluent spectrum to show formation of fluorescing DOM

LC-OCD (DOC-LABOR, Germany) analysis of the samples for MR, MR+SOM, SE and CR were performed. Five distinguishable peaks appeared in the LC-OCD chromatograms that are characteristic of organic carbon fractions: (i) biopolymers, (ii) humic substances, (iii) building block, (iv) neutrals and (v) low molecular weight (MW) acids. Each fraction was determined from the chromatogram, representing a concentration of organic carbon (Figure 5.10 and Table 5.4). LC-OCD showed an almost complete removal of biopolymers (MW > 20,000-dalton) for all samples because the biopolymer fraction is mainly comprised of biodegradable organic matter in the form of proteins and polysaccharides.

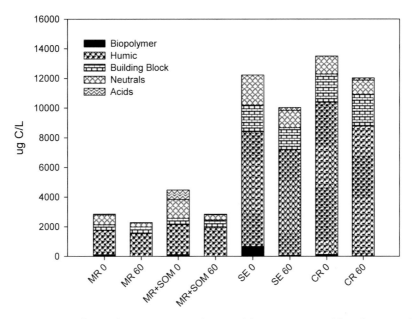

Figure 5.10 Organic carbon concentrations with respect to biopolymers, humic substances, building blocks, neutrals and acids using LC-OCD during batch study with different types of water under biotic conditions (contact time: 60 days)

Table 5.4 Summary of organic carbon concentrations with respect to biopolymers, humic substances, building blocks, neutrals and acids using LC-OCD

	Biopolymer (ug/L)	Humic (ug/L)	Building Block (ug/L)	Neutrals (ug/L)	Low MW acids (ug/L)
MR 0	100	1663	373	667	53
MR 60	13	1541	431	268	29
MR+SOM 0	104	2045	421	1256	650
MR+SOM 60	11	1950	495	354	39
SE 0	653	7755	1790	2033	0
SE 60	60	7133	1479	1165	187
CR 0	122	10272	1890	1212	0
CR 60	27	8748	2148	951	148

After 60 days of contact time, LC-OCD showed a similar removal trend in organic matter fractions for MR and MR+SOM reactors. MR and MR+SOM reactors used the same source of water (e.g., The Meuse River) except that MR+SOM contained an additional external carbon source (i.e., SOM). This additional carbon source also appeared in LC-OCD chromatograms which led to higher concentrations in acids and neutral fractions (Figure 5.10). About 1.5 mg/L and 2 mg/L of humic substances were detected in the MR and the MR+SOM samples after 60 days of contact time, respectively. A slightly higher fraction of humic substances was measured in the MR+SOM compared to the MR, and the SUVA of the MR+SOM (SUVA = 4.72 L/mg-m) was also higher than that of the MR (SUVA = 4.26 L/mg-m). This slight increase in humic fraction and SUVA could also correspond to the formation of fluorescing DOM (i.e., humic-like peak) from the F-EEM spectra observed. Jarusutthirak and Amy (2007) observed the transformation of organic compounds during biological processes using glucose as a sole carbon source for bacterial growth and showed the transformation of glucose (MW: 180-dalton) to a higher MW organic matter during a biological process. Therefore, the biodegradation of labile organic matter (e.g., low MW glucose) in the MR+SOM could be attributed to the formation of fluorescing humic substances (P2) and humic fraction (MW > 350-dalton).

SE showed a fairly high concentration of biopolymers (MW >20,000-dalton) compared to MR, MR+SOM and CR because of soluble microbial products (SMPs) present in SE (Figure 5.10). SMPs are part of the biopolymer containing polysaccharide- and protein-like substances. SMPs are biologically derived products from substrate metabolism during the growth of biomass in a biological wastewater treatment process (Jarusutthirak and Amy, 2007). In contrast, the removal of DOC from the CR mainly occurred in the humic substances fraction according to the LC-OCD analysis, and this removal can be better explained by adsorption than biodegradation due to the refractory properties of humic substances in the CR. Moreover, AMB measured by ATP in the CR was also lower than that of the MR and the MR+SOM, suggesting biodegradation was relatively low and did not contribute significantly to the removal of DOC.

The primary mechanism in the removal of dissolved organic matter during RBF is biodegradation by partial biotransformation or complete mineralization (Shamrukh and Abdel-Wahab, 2008). After 60 days of contact time, AMB measured as ATP concentrations associated with sand for NCTW, SE, MR+SOM, MR and CR were 2.1, 10.2, 7.9, 6.4 and 4.5 ng ATP/cm^3, respectively. The ATP concentrations associated with sand were relatively low compared to sands from slow sand filters operating in three different water treatment plants in the Netherlands (i.e., 18 - 93 ng ATP/cm^3, Magic-Knezev and van der Kooij, 2004)). This was due limited carbon sources and nutrients during long residence time (60 days). However, their average ATP concentrations were still correlated to the amount of BDOC concentrations introduced into batch reactors except for CR. In the CR, BDOC measured as an average DOC removal during 60 days was higher than that from MR and MR+SOM, however, the ATP concentration associated with sand from the CR was relatively low. This result implies that DOC was not utilized for energy or microbial growth by microorganisms, and rather was just adsorbed onto sand. Also, the low ATP concentration observed in the CR also corresponds to LC-OCD results in that the humic fraction was mainly removed during 60 days of contact time, suggesting biodegradation was relatively low and did not significantly to microbial growth. Trulleyov and Rul (2004) showed that there is a certain overestimation in BDOC results if some part of adsorbed DOC is resistant to biodegradation. This could be the case for the CR in this study. A comparison between ATP concentrations and DOC reductions for the different water types suggested that there was an overestimation of BDOC results for the CR. A slight increase in SUVA, relatively low transformation of organic matter (F-EEM), and low AMB in the CR also support the refractory characteristics of DOM. Therefore, BDOC measured as an average removal of DOC may not be applicable to represent the amount of organic matter utilized by microorganisms when a sample contains a high content of humic substances.

5.3.2. Pharmaceutically active compounds

In batch reactors, selected neutral PhACs with low K_{ow} (log K_{ow} < 2, Table 5.1) (phenacetine, paracetamol and caffeine) and acidic PhACs (ibuprofen, fenoprofen and naproxen) exhibited removal efficiencies greater than 87% from different water types with respect to BDOC and humic contents (i.e., different organic matter characteristics) during 60 days of contact time (Table 5.5). These compounds are mostly analgesics except for caffeine. However, removal efficiencies for gemfibrozil and clofibric acid (i.e., lipid regulators) were low. Such low removal efficiencies might be caused by biodiversity in microorganisms, carbon limitation during co-metabolism or adsorption competition between humic substances and selected PhACs. Moreover, removal efficiencies of diclofenac, gemfibrozil and clofibric acid from batch reactors containing non-chlorinated tap water (NCTW) significantly decreased to 9.8%, 28%, and 0%, respectively. NCTW had less humic substances (i.e., less potential competition between humic substances and PhACs for binding sites) and a low BDOC concentration compared to that of the other water types. Thus, the adsorption capacity of PhACs in NCTW may be greater than in the other batch reactors which may lead to more favorable conditions for selected PhACs to adsorb onto sand. However, the removal efficiencies of diclofenac, gemfibrozil and clofibric acid were low in NCTW which implied that removal efficiencies depended on the amount of BDOC available. Therefore, co-metabolism may play an important role in the removal of diclofenac, gemfibrozil and clofibric acid. Lim et al. (2008) showed that biotransformation rates of some PhACs (e.g., diclofenac and gemfibrozil) increased as initial concentration of BDOC in wastewater increased. This result suggests that the amount of BDOC is related to the removal of PhACs. On the other hand, neutral PhACs with low K_{ow} (log K_{ow} < 0.3, Table 5.1) compounds like paracetamol, phenacetine and caffeine were removed even in the NCTW. BDOC concentration estimated in the NCTW was only 0.5 mg/L, and similar results were also obtained in column studies described in the latter part of this study.

Table 5.5 Removal efficiencies of wastewater-derived compounds during batch experiments (contact time: 60 days)

Compound	Removal (%)					
	SE	CR	MR+SOM	MR	TAP	Blank
Gemfibrozil	76	44	83	86	28	2
Diclofenac	83	65	97	94	9.8	0
Ibuprofen	97	96	97	94	98	13
Fenoprofen	92	92	93	88	94	0
Bezafibrate	98	97	98	94	91	21
Ketoprofen	97	97	97	94	21	4
Naproxen	97	97	98	95	94	29
Clofibric acid	84	63	46	66	0	0
Carbamazepine	0	0	0	0	0	0
Phenacetine	97	97	98	98	97	0
Pentoxifylline	97	97	89	94	50	16
Paracetamol	96	91	98	97	96	0
Caffeine	97	96	98	97	96	0

Among PhACs analyzed, carbamazepine (i.e., an anticonvulsant) was the most persistent compound and not influenced by different organic matter characteristics. According to previous studies, carbamazepine has shown a persistent behavior in the environment, and the removal is less than 10% in most wastewater treatment plants (Stamatelatou et al., 2003; Ternes, 1998; Ternes et al., 2004; Zhang et al., 2008). Clara et al. (2004) proposed carbamazepine as a tracer for anthropogenic influences in the aquatic environment.

5.3.3. Comparison of biodegradation and sorption for selected PhAC removals

Dissolved organic matter characteristics

Table 5.6 summarizes pH, DOC, SUVA and ATP concentrations for column studies. The average DOC of NCTW was 1.95 mg/L which decreased to 1.50 during column studies with average removal of 23%. Like the batch reactor experiments mentioned earlier, the increase in SUVA for MR columns (SC2 and SC3) also indicated the preferential removal of aliphatic organic matter. DOC removal for the SC4 (DW + NaN$_3$) was less than 0.02 mg/L which is mainly attributable to the level of experimental error. The detection limit of the TOC analyzer used in this study was 0.05 mg/L; thus the removal efficiencies observed from the SC4 (DW + NaN$_3$) were negligible. ATP concentrations associated with sand were measured to ensure that all columns were operated under biotic (SC1, SC2 and SC3) or abiotic (SC4) conditions. Average ATP concentrations associated with sand for column depths between 10 mm and 290 mm were 30, 102, and 0.6 g ATP/cm^3 for SC1, SC2, and SC4, respectively by the end of the experiment (e.g., 60 days of operation).

Table 5.6 Summary of characteristics for influent and effluent from SC1, SC2, SC3 and SC4 after acclimation

	Time (day)	pH	DOC (mg/L)	BDOC (mg/L)	Average ATP (ATP/cm^3)	SUVA (L/mg-m)
SC1	0	7.63	1.95	0.45	30	2.46
(NCTW)	1.2	8.09	1.50			2.34
SC2	0	7.95	5.94	3.2	102	2.90
(MR)	1.2	8.26	2.74			3.27
SC3	0	7.98	5.19	2.82	-	2.43
(MR)	1.2	8.26	2.37			3.08
SC4,	0	6.80	1.31	0.02	0.6	13.03
(DW+NaN$_3$)	1.2	7.23	1.29			13.50

Figures 5.11, 5.12, 5.13 and 5.14 present F-EEM for SC1, SC2, SC3 and SC4, respectively. Figure 5.11 shows that there was no reduction in FI for P1 and P2, while the FI for P3 was reduced by 38% in NCTW (SC1). The removal of FI for P3 was an indication of some protein-like substances present in the NCTW. However, the FI of P3 in the NCTW was relatively small compared to that of other samples. Moreover, FI intensities for P1, P2 and P3 were relatively low in the NCTW because of low organic matter. Figure 5.12 exhibited 9%, 34.4%, and 54.5% removals for P1, P2 and P3, respectively, for SC2 (MR, 60 days acclimation). Figure 5.13 exhibited 7.7%, 8.7% and 24.5% removals for P1, P2 and P3, respectively, for the MR column acclimated for 10 days (SC3). SC2 and SC3 showed high FI for P3 compared to the NCTW. Figure 5.14 shows that FI changes for SC4 (abiotic conditions, DW+NaN$_3$), and F-EEM spectra observed under abiotic conditions did not change. A very low FI for P3 in SC4 may be contributed by PhACs that have fluorescing structures. F-EEM spectra observed in SC4 were substantially lower than those for SC2 and SC3; thus, the FI reduction in SC4 was negligible as result of very low DOC and in the presence of a biocide in SC4.

114

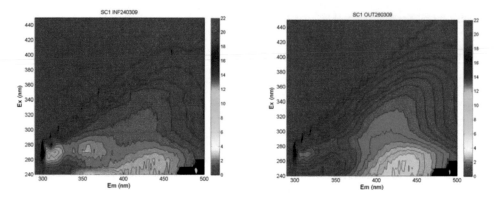

Figure 5.11 F-EEM spectra of SC1 fed with NCTW (a) influent and (b) effluent (EBCT: 11-hr)

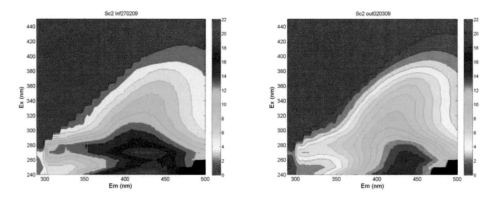

Figure 5.12 F-EEM spectra of SC2 fed with MR (a) influent and (b) effluent (EBCT: 11-hr)

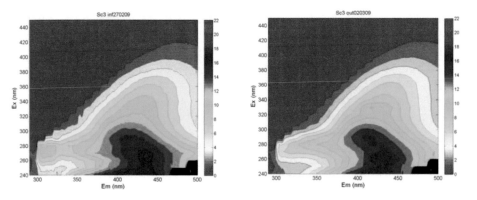

Figure 5.13 F-EEM spectra of SC3 fed with MR: (a) influent and (b) effluent (EBCT: 11-hr, 10-day acclimation period)

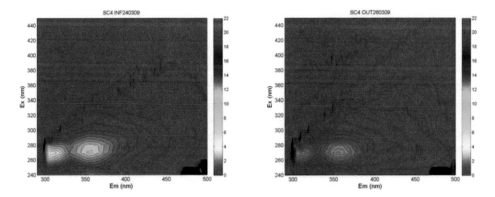

Figure 5.14 F-EEM spectra of SC4 fed with demineralized water with sodium azide: (a) influent and (b) effluent (EBCT: 11-hr)

Figure 5.15 and Table 5.7 show the LC-OCD results of SC1, SC2, SC3 and SC4. Biopolymers defined by LC-OCD for SC1 and SC2 were removed 83% and 57%, respectively. The humic substances fraction in NCTW was relatively low, and these results corresponded to the F-EEM spectra where P1 and P2 were also low. Even though different acclimation times were provided for SC2 (60 days) and SC3 (10 days), the removals in different organic matter fractions were similar between SC2 and SC3 after 60 days of operation. ATP concentrations associated with sand from SC2 and SC3 were 102 and 91 g ATP/cm^3, respectively. AMB measurement requires dismantling a column to take sand samples, thus samples from SC3 were taken after 60 days of operation which lead to AMB in SC3 close to that of SC2. For SC4, the humic substances fraction was not detected by LC-OCD, and there was no change in organic matter fractions during the time of the study.

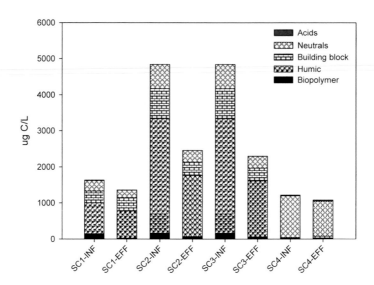

Figure 5.15 The change of organic matter fractions (biopolymers, humic substances, building blocks, neutrals and low MW acids) determined by LC-OCD for SC1, SC2, SC3 and SC4

Table 5.7 Summary of organic carbon concentrations with respect to biopolymers, humic substances, building blocks, neutrals and acids using LC-OCD

	Biopolymer (ug/L)	Humic (ug/L)	Building Block (ug/L)	Neutrals (ug/L)	Low MW acids (ug/L)
MR 0	146	854	326	294	10
MR 60	25	755	365	208	5
MR+SOM 0	164	3168	838	671	2
MR+SOM 60	70	1690	377	321	0
SE 0	164	3168	838	671	2
SE 60	58	1553	357	328	2
CR 0	12	0	29	1155	22
CR 60	19	0	59	971	33

Pharmaceutically active compounds

Figure 5.16 shows that removal efficiencies of phenacetine, pentoxifylline, caffeine and pentoxifylline (i.e., hydrophilic-neutral, log K_{ow} < 2) were above 91% for SC2 (60 days acclimated column). However, for SC3, the short acclimation time (i.e., 10 days) decreased removal efficiencies of phenacetine and pentoxifylline by 14% and 31%, respectively. Moreover, removal efficiencies of gemfibrozil, diclofenac and fenoprofen (acidic PhACs) were 35%, 20% and 78% for SC2 (60 days acclimated column) and 0%, 5% and 42% for SC3 (10 days acclimated column), respectively. This implies that the removals of these compounds correlate with microbial activity (ATP) associated with the sand.

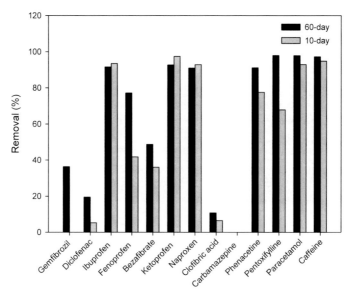

Figure 5.16 Impact of acclimation period on the removal of wastewater-derived compounds (SC2 (60 days) and SC3 (10 days), EBCT: 11 hours)

However, at the same time, the organic carbon content associated with the sand could be different due to the different acclimation period; thus, removal efficiencies observed for hydrophobic compounds (e.g., gemfibrozil, diclofenac and fenoprofen) could be affected by different organic carbon contents associated with the sand. Therefore, an additional experiment was carried out using SC1 and SC2 columns, which had the same acclimation time (i.e., approximately the same organic carbon content) to determine the impact of low microbial activity by introducing low BDOC water (e.g., NCTW). In addition, the role of BDOC in the removal of PhACs was also determined from SC1 and SC2. After 2 months of acclimation with MR, the feed water to SC1 was changed from MR to NCTW (i.e., low BDOC). BDOC concentrations for NCTW (SC1) and MR (SC2) were 0.45 mg/L and 3.2 mg/L, respectively. Low BDOC in NCTW resulted in low microbial activity over the first 50 mm of SC1 (ATP = 30 ng ATP/cm^3) compared to that of MR (SC2, ATP = 102 ng ATP/cm^3). Removal efficiencies of acidic PhACs (i.e., analgesics) decreased as result of low BDOC (Figure 5.17). However, hydrophilic neutral compounds such as paracetamol, pentoxifylline, phenacetine and caffeine were still removed above 91% in SC1. Microorganisms appear to be still capable of removing paracetamol, pentoxifylline, phenacetine and caffeine in NCTW, possibly by direct as opposed to co-metabolism. In order to define if these compounds were removed by biodegradation in NCTW, an abiotic experiment was necessary to examine the PhACs removals by sorption.

In SC4 (abiotic conditions), removal efficiencies of hydrophilic neutral PhACs (paracetamol, pentoxifylline, phenacetine and caffeine) were less than 17% and significantly decreased because of abiotic conditions (Figure 5.17). These substantially low removal efficiencies observed in SC4 were attributed to inactivation of microorganisms by sodium azide; thus, such hydrophilic neutral PhACs easily passed through the column. This implies that the dominant removal mechanism for these compounds was biodegradation. An average removal of 30% was observed for acidic PhACs under abiotic conditions. The pH of influent and effluent samples ranged between 7.63 and 8.19, and the pH range tested in this study was higher than the pK_a of selected acidic PhACs. Removal efficiencies of hydrophobic ionic compounds (log D at pH 8 greater than > 1) such as gemfibrozil, diclofenac, ibuprofen and fenoprofen may have decreased due to electrostatic interactions under abiotic conditions. However, under biotic conditions, removal efficiencies of these compounds were significantly increased (i.e., SC2). These results confirmed the importance of biodegradation for PhAC removal during soil passage.

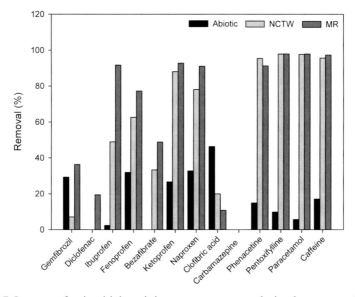

Figure 5.17 Impact of microbial activity on wastewater-derived compounds (Abiotic conditions: SC4, NCTW: SC1 and MR: SC2, EBCT: 11 hours)

5.4. Conclusions

Based on the results obtained in this study, the following conclusions can be drawn:

- The formation of humic-like fluorescing DOM was observed as result of extended biodegradation (i.e., 60 days combined oxic (30 days) and anoxic (30 days) conditions) by F-EEM, and this is part of transformation of DOM during biodegradation.

- Biopolymers degraded more favorably compared to other fractions of DOM according to LC-OCD, and active microbial biomass associated with sand determined by ATP reflected the availability of BDOC.

- Neutral PhACs (phenacetine, pentoxifylline, paracetamol and caffeine) and acidic PhACs (ibuprofen, fenoprofen, bezafibrate, ketoprofen and naproxen) exhibited removal efficiencies of greater than 87% from different types of waters during batch studies (contact time: 60 days).

- Removals efficiencies of phenacetine, pentoxifylline, gemfibrozil, bezafibrate and fenoprofen increased with acclimation time.

- Removal efficiencies of acidic PhACs (i.e., analgesics) decreased under biodegradable carbon limited conditions. This implies that co-metabolism may play important role in the removal of acidic PhACs.

- Removal efficiencies of acidic PhACs (ibuprofen, fenoprofen, ketoprofen and naproxen) and hydrophilic neutral PhACs (paracetamol, pentoxifylline, phenacetine and caffeine) with low K_{ow} (log K_{ow} < 2) were less than 35% under abiotic conditions. However, removal efficiencies of these compounds were greater 78% under biotic conditions, and this is mainly attributed to biodegradation.

- Hydrophilic neutral PhACs (paracetamol, pentoxifylline, phenacetine and caffeine) were still removed under carbon limited conditions, suggesting that these compounds may have been used as a carbon source (i.e., direct metabolism) for microorganism growth.

- Carbamazepine showed a persistent behavior under both biotic and abiotic conditions.

- Results of this study showed that biodegradation is an important mechanism for removing PhACs during soil passage. This implies that when properly designed and operated, removal of PhACs during RBF is a sustainable treatment option.

5.5. References

Amy, G. and Drewes, J., 2007. Soil Aquifer Treatment (SAT) as Natural and Sustainable Wastewater Reclamation/Reuse Technology: Fate of Wastewater Effluent Organic Matter (EfOM) and Trace Organic Compounds. Environ. Monit. Assess., 129(1-3), 19-26.

Boxall, A.B.A., Kay, P., Blackwell, P.A. and Fogg, L.A., 2004. Fate of Veterinary Medicines Applied to Soils. Pharmaceuticals in the Environment. Springer, Berlin.

Cha, W., Choi, H., Kim, J. and Kim, I.S., 2004. Evaluation of wastewater effluents for soil aquifer treatment in South Korea. Water Sci. Technol., 50(2), 315-322.

Chen, H., Chen, S., Quan, X., Zhao, H. and Zhang, Y., 2008. Sorption of polar and nonpolar organic contaminants by oil-contaminated soil. Chemosphere, 73(11), 1832-1837.

Clara, M., Strenn, B. and Kreuzinger, N., 2004. Carbamazepine as a possible anthropogenic marker in the aquatic environment: investigations on the behaviour of Carbamazepine in wastewater treatment and during groundwater infiltration. Water Res., 38(4), 947-954.

Coble, P.G., 1996. Characterization of marine and terrestrial DOM in seawater using excitation-emission matrix spectroscopy. Mar. Chem., 51(4), 325-346.

Cunningham, V.L., 2004. Special Characteristics of Pharmaceuticals related to Environmental Fate. Pharmaceuticals in the Environment. Springer, Berlin.

Grünheid, S. and Jekel, M., 2005. Fate of trace organic pollutants during bank filtration and groundwater recharge, Proceeding of 5th International Symposium on Management of Aquifer Recharge, 10-16 June 2005, Berlin, Germany.

Heberer, T., 2002. Occurrence, fate, and removal of pharmaceutical residues in the aquatic environment: a review of recent research data. Toxicol. Lett., 131(1-2), 5-17.

Heberer, T. et al., 2004. Field Studies on the Fate and Transport of Pharmaceutical Residues in Bank Filtration. Ground Water Monit. R., 24(2), 70-77.

Henderson, R.K. et al., 2009. Fluorescence as a potential monitoring tool for recycled water systems: A review. Water Res., 43(4), 863-881.

Howard, P.H., 2000. Biodegradation. Handbook of Property Estimation Methods for Chemicals: Environmental Health Sciences CRC Press LLC, Boca Raton.

Huber, S. and Frimmel, F.H., 1992. A liquid chromatographic system with multi-detection for the direct analysis of hydrophilic organic compounds in natural waters. Fresenius' J. Anal. Chem., 342(1-2), 198-200.

Hudson, N. et al., 2008. Can fluorescence spectrometry be used as a surrogate for the Biochemical Oxygen Demand (BOD) test in water quality assessment? An example from South West England., Sci. Total Environ., 391(1), 149-158.

Jarusutthirak, C. and Amy, G., 2007. Understanding soluble microbial products (SMP) as a component of effluent organic matter (EfOM). Water Res., 41(12), 2787-2793.

Jjemba, P.K., 2006. Excretion and ecotoxicity of pharmaceutical and personal care products in the environment. Ecotox. Environ. Safe., 63(1), 113-130.

Kim, S.D., Cho, J., Kim, I.S., Vanderford, B.J. and Snyder, S.A., 2007. Occurrence and removal of pharmaceuticals and endocrine disruptors in South Korean surface, drinking, and waste waters. Water Res., 41(5), 1013-1021.

Kümmerer, K., 2009. The presence of pharmaceuticals in the environment due to human use - present knowledge and future challenges. J. Environ. Manage., 90(8), 2354-2366.

Leenheer, J.A. and Croue, J.-P., 2003. Characterizing aquatic dissolved organic matter. Environ. Sci. Technol., 37(1), 18A-26A.

Liang, C., Dang, Z., Xiao, B., Huang, W. and Liu, C., 2006. Equilibrium sorption of phenanthrene by soil humic acids. Chemosphere, 63(11), 1961-1968.

Lim, M.-H., Snyder, S.A. and Sedlak, D.L., 2008. Use of biodegradable dissolved organic carbon (BDOC) to assess the potential for transformation of wastewater-derived contaminants in surface waters. Water Res., 42(12), 2943-2952.

Madden, J.C., Enoch, S.J., Hewitt, M. and Cronin, M.T.D., 2009. Pharmaceuticals in the environment: Good practice in predicting acute ecotoxicological effects. Toxicol. Lett., 185(2), 85-101.

Maeng, S.K., Sharma, S.K., Amy, G. and Magic-Knezev, A., 2008. Fate of effluent organic matter (EfOM) and natural organic matter (NOM) through riverbank filtration. Water Sci. Technol., 57(12), 1999–2007.

Magic-Knezev, A. and van der Kooij, D., 2004. Optimisation and significance of ATP analysis for measuring active biomass in granular activated carbon filters used in water treatment. Water Res., 38(18), 3971-3979.

Massmann, G., Dunnbier, U., Heberer, T. and Taute, T., 2008. Behaviour and redox sensitivity of pharmaceutical residues during bank filtration - Investigation of residues of phenazone-type analgesics. Chemosphere, 71(8), 1476-1485.

Mechlinski, A. and Heberer, T., 2005. Fate and transport of pharmaceutical residues during bank filtration, Proceeding of ISMAR 2005, Berlin, 542-547.

Mompelat, S., LeBot, B. and Thomas, O., 2009. Occurrence and fate of pharmaceutical products and by-products, from resource to drinking water. Environ. Int., 35, 803-814.

Oades, J.M. and Jenkinson, D.S., 1979. Adenosine triphosphate content of the soil microbial biomass. Soil Biol. Biochem., 11(2), 201-204.

Ogawa, H., Amagai, Y., Koike, I., Kaiser, K. and Benner, R., 2001. Production of refractory dissolved organic matter by bacteria. Science, 292, 917-920.

Saadi, I., Borisover, M., Armon, R. and Laor, Y., 2006. Monitoring of effluent DOM biodegradation using fluorescence, UV and DOC measurements. Chemosphere, 63(3), 530-539.

Sacher, F., Ehmann, M., Gabriel, S., Graf, C. and Brauch, H.-J., 2008. Pharmaceutical residues in the river Rhine-Results of a one-decade monitoring programme., J. Environ. Monit., 10, 664-670.

Schmidt, C.K., Lange, F.T. and Brauch, H.J., 2007. Characteristics and evaluation of natural attenuation processes for organic micropollutant removal during riverbank filtration, Proceeding of regional IWA Conference on Groundwater Management in the Danube river Basin and other Large River Basins, Belgrade, 231-236.

Shamrukh, M. and Abdel-Wahab, A., 2008. Riverbank filtration for sustainable water supply: application to a large-scale facility on the Nile River. Clean Technol. Envir., 10(4), 351-358.

Snyder, S.A. et al., 2004. Biological and Physical Attenuation of Endocrine Disruptors and Pharmaceuticals: Implications for Water Reuse. Ground Water Monit. R., 24(2), 108-118.

Stamatelatou, K. et al., 2003. Pharmaceuticals and health care products in wastewater effluents: the example of carbamazepine. Water Sci. Technol., 3, 131-137.

US EPA, 2009. Estimation Programs Interface Suite™ for Microsoft® Windows, v 4.00. United States Environmental Protection Agency, Washington, DC, USA.

Ternes, T.A., 1998. Occurrence of drugs in German sewage treatment plants and rivers. Water Res., 32(11), 3245-3260.

Ternes, T.A. et al., 2004. A rapid method to measure the solid-water distribution coefficient (Kd) for pharmaceuticals and musk fragrances in sewage sludge. Water Res., 38(19), 4075-4084.

Trulleyov, S.k. and Rul, M., 2004. Determination of biodegradable dissolved organic carbon in waters: comparison of batch methods. Sci. Total Environ., 332(1-3), 253-260.

Urfer, D. and Huck, P.M., 2001. Measurement of biomass activity in drinking water biofilters using a respirometric method. Water Res., 35(6), 1469-1477.

Xue, S., Zhao, Q.-L., Wei, L.-L. and Ren, N.-Q., 2009. Behavior and characteristics of dissolved organic matter during column studies of soil aquifer treatment. Water Res., 43(2), 499-507.

Yangali-Quintanilla, V., Sadmani, A., McConville, M., Kennedy, M., Amy, G., 2010. A QSAR model for predicting rejection of emerging contaminants (pharmaceuticals, endocrine disruptors) by nanofiltration membranes. Water Res., 44(2), 373-384.

Zhang, Y., Geissen, S.-U. and Gal, C., 2008. Carbamazepine and diclofenac: Removal in wastewater treatment plants and occurrence in water bodies. Chemosphere, 73(8), 1151-1161.

Chapter 6

ORGANIC MICROPOLLUUTANT REMOVAL FROM WASTEWATER EFFLUENT-IMPACTED DRINKING WATER SOURCES DURING BANK FILTRATION AND ARTIFICIAL RECHARGE

Parts of this chapter were based on:

Maeng, S.K., Ameda, E.A., Sharma, S.K., Grützmacher, G. and Amy, G.L., 2010. Organic micropollutant removal from wastewater effluent-impacted drinking water sources during bank filtration and artificial recharge. Water Research, 44 (11), 4003-4014.

124

Summary

Natural treatment systems such as bank filtration (BF) and artificial recharge (via an infiltration basin) are robust barriers for many organic micropollutants (OMPs) and may represent a low-cost alternative compared to advanced drinking water treatment systems. This study analyzes a comprehensive database of OMPs at BF and artificial recharge (AR) sites located near Lake Tegel in Berlin (Germany). The focus of the study was on the derivation of correlations between the removal efficiencies of OMPs and key factors influencing the performance of BF and AR. At the BF site, shallow monitoring wells located close to the Lake Tegel source exhibited oxic conditions followed by prolonged anoxic conditions in deep monitoring wells and a production well. At the AR site, oxic conditions prevailed from the recharge pond along monitoring wells to the production well. Long residence times of up to 4.5 months at the BF site reduced the temperature variation during soil passage between summer and winter. The temperature variations were greater at the AR site as a consequence of shorter residence times. Deep monitoring wells and the production well located at the BF site were under the influence of ambient groundwater and *old* bank filtrate (up to several years of age). Thus, it is important to account for mixing with native groundwater and other sources (e.g., old bank filtrate) when estimating the performance of BF with respect to removal of OMPs. At the BF site, principal component analysis (PCA) was used to investigate correlations between OMP removals and hydrogeochemical conditions with spatial and temporal parameters (e.g., well distance, residence time and depth) from both sites. Principal component-1 (PC1) embodied redox conditions (oxidation reduction potential and dissolved oxygen), and principal component-2 (PC2) embodied degradation potential (e.g., total organic carbon and dissolved organic carbon) and the calcium carbonate dissolution potential (Ca^{2+} and HCO_3^-) for the BF site. These two PCs explained a total variance of 55% at the BF site. At the AR site, PCA revealed redox conditions (PC1) and degradation potential with temperature (PC2) as principal components, which explained a total variance of 56%.

6.1. Introduction

Organic micropollutants (OMPs) including pharmaceutically active compounds (PhACs), endocrine disrupting compounds (EDCs) and personal care products (PCPs) are increasingly being identified in the environment due to development of analytical technologies with lower detection limits (Snyder et al., 2004). Human pharmaceuticals are used to cure patients and protect people from diseases (Cunningham et al., 2006). However, several pharmaceuticals and metabolites from patient excretion in wastewater are not removed by conventional wastewater treatment processes (Heberer, 2002a, b; Kim et al., 2007). Although PhACs and their transformation products are present in aquatic environments, scientists have shown that at low (ng/L) levels, individual PhACs do not pose an appreciable risk to human health (Schwab, 2005). However, the possible detrimental effects of *mixtures* of EDCs, PhACs and PCPs on the aquatic environment and lifelong exposure to humans are currently unknown, especially for recently developed chemicals (Halling-Soensen et al., 1998; Cunningham et al., 2006).

Bank filtration (BF) and artificial recharge (AR) (i.e., infiltration basin), as managed aquifer recharge (MAR) processes, are reliable and proven natural water treatment systems (Irmscher and Teermann, 2002). In Europe, there are many cities that have implemented BF or AR as one of the main steps for drinking water treatment (Grünheid et al., 2005; Jekel and Grünheid, 2005; Eckert and Irmscher, 2006). It is important to investigate the natural attenuation of OMPs during BF and AR in order to determine the post-treatment requirements for residues of OMPs, more systematically. This is a crucial design aspect for new water treatment plants with BF or AR or for existing plants that are considering retrofit for advanced treatment processes to remove OMPs.

The objective of this study was to compare the removal efficiencies of selected OMPs at BF and AR sites in Berlin and investigate correlations between OMP removals, hydrogeochemical conditions, and spatial parameters (e.g., well distances, residence times and depths). In a first step OMP data from field-based studies at BF and AR sites were compiled and analyzed by integrating information that had not been available before, e.g., mixing (for details concerning sampling and chemical analysis refer to Massmann et al. (2008) and Zuehlke et al. (2007)). Together with this additional information the selected OMPs and hydrogeochemical parameters (e.g., redox potential, dissolved oxygen, pH, Fe, Mn, etc.) were then analyzed using principal component analysis (PCA) in order to statistically delineate removal trends at BF and AR sites.

6.2. Field sites and research methodology

The NASRI project (2002-2005) of KWB Berlin (Germany) investigated geochemical processes and hydrogeology as well as the fate of pathogens, algal toxins (not discussed herein), and OMPs at BF and AR sites (Figure 6.1). This study included data from the BF and AR sites: Lake Tegel BF site and Lake Tegel AR site (Tegel water works, pond 3). The BF and AR sites are managed by the Berlin Water Works (Berliner Wasserbetriebe, BWB), which supplies drinking water for 3.7 million people in the city of Berlin. Approximately, 22% of the Lake Tegel water at the Lake Tegel BF site originated from treated wastewater effluent from the Schönerlinde wastewater treatment plant (Pekdeger, 2006).

126

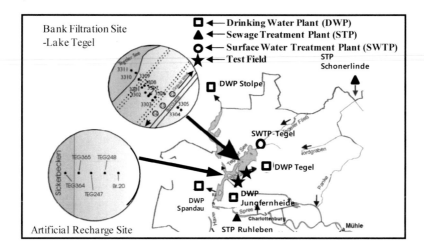

Figure 6.1. NASRI BF and AR transects at Lake Tegel field site (modified and reproduced from Fritz (2003)).

6.2.1. Bank filtration site – Lake Tegel

The Lake Tegel BF site consists of 8 shallow monitoring wells, 5 deep monitoring wells, 1 ambient groundwater monitoring well and 1 production well. Locations of the monitoring wells and the production well are shown in Figure 6.2. A background well (number 3304) showed 100% groundwater and was monitored for comparing background groundwater quality with bank filtrate (Grünheid et al., 2005; Pekdeger, 2006). Data from well TEG374, which is the deepest well among the rest of the monitoring wells, was used in the analysis to differentiate old bank filtrate which originates from the deeper sections of the upper aquifer. Pekdeger (2006) estimated that the residence time of the old bank filtrate is approximately a decade by a radioactive isotope of hydrogen (T/3He). As our study focused on OMP concentrations for young bank filtrate (maximum residence time 4.5-months), the impacts of mixing with groundwater and old bank filtrate were taken into account while analyzing the removal efficiencies of OMPs in the bank filtrate. For example, 1-Acetyl-1-methyl-2-dimethyl-oxymoyl-2-phenylhydrazide (AMDOPH) was observed to be significantly higher in the old bank filtrate than in the young bank filtrate at the BF site. AMDOPH is a metabolite of phenazone-type pharmaceuticals (dimethylaminophenazone), and it is known as a persistent pharmaceutical compound in the environment (Zuehlke et al., 2007). Occurrence of AMDOPH in the old bank filtrate from the BF site has been reported to be due to discharge from a former pharmaceutical production plant located north-west of Berlin, in the former East Germany where they produced phenazone-type pharmaceuticals which may have been discharged into the Havel river (Reddersen et al., 2002). In analysis of the data, corrections for the mixing from the groundwater and the old bank filtrate were made for the wells with young bank filtrate proportions that were less than 100%. Therefore, the deep monitoring wells and the production well No. 13, where the young bank filtrate proportions were less than 100%, were corrected for mixing effects. The mixing effect from the groundwater increased with respect to the vertical and horizontal distances from Lake Tegel. The correction for mixing was carried out using a mass balance (based on AMDOPH) of the reported well concentration measurements as given below:

$$C_{Well} = (\%_{Young\,bank\,filtrate} \times C_{Young\,bank\,filtrate}) + (\%_{Native\,groundwater} \times C_{Groundwater}) + (\%_{Old\,bank\,filtrate} \times C_{Old\,bank\,filtrate})$$

$$\text{Hence, } C_{Young\,bank\,filtrate} = \frac{C_{well} - (\%_{Groundwater} \times C_{Groundwater}) - (\%_{Old\,bank\,filtrate} \times C_{Old\,bank\,filtrate})}{\%_{Young\,bank\,filtrate}} ..$$

(1)

%: relative share (between 0 and 100%),

C: observed or calculated concentration of a certain substance (µg/L)

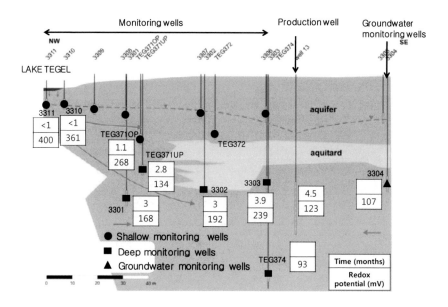

Figure 6.2 Cross-section of BF site showing the well locations and the flow paths to a production well (modified and adopted from Pekdeger (2006) and Massmann et al. (2006))

6.2.2. Artificial recharge site (infiltration basin)

The artificial groundwater recharge site studied in the NASRI project consists of a recharge (infiltration) pond (recharge pond No.3), 10 monitoring wells, 3 groundwater monitoring wells and the production well No.20, with the site located near the eastern bank of Lake Tegel. Figure 6.3 shows a cross section of the AR site. Lake Tegel water, abstracted from the southern part of the Lake, was pumped into the pond and recharged into the aquifer comprised of fine to middle grained sands of hydraulic conductivity 2 – 8×10^{-4} m/s (Pekdeger, 2006). In contrast to the BF site, the infiltrates flowing from the recharge pond to all monitoring wells are reported to be purely *young* recharged water, and the proportion of groundwater in abstracted water from the production No. 20 was 20% (Grünheid et al., 2005). Further details are given in Greskowiak et al. (2005).

The hydraulic flow paths of the bank filtrate from Lake Tegel towards the production well No. 13, postulated by Pekdeger (2006) and Massmann et al. (2006), are shown by the arrows in Figure 6.3. The flow of the bank filtrate traverses a short oxic zone in the shallow monitoring wells (3311, 3310, TEG371OP and TEG372) section on its way to the deeper monitoring wells (TEG371UP, 3301, 3302 and 3303) that are mainly in an anoxic zone. Previous studies have given more detailed information on the transect of the Lake Tegel site (Heberer et al., 2004; Grünheid et al., 2005; Jekel and Grünheid, 2005).

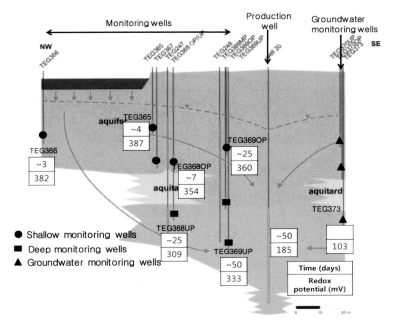

Figure 6.3 Cross-section of AR site showing the well locations and the flow paths to the production well (modified and adopted from Pekdeger (2006) and Massmann et al. (2006))

6.2.3. Data treatment and principal component analysis

Prior to performing PCA, data sets from the BF and AR sites were standardized in order to eliminate the influence of wide variation in measurements with different units and to ensure that each variable is equally weighted. The standardization was applied to all data sets by first subtracting the mean and dividing by the standard deviation (s) from each data set (Cloutier et al., 2008). After standardization of original data X_i, new standardized values Z_i have a mean and variance of zero and 1, respectively ($Z_i = (X_i-$ mean)/s) (Davis, 1986). The data obtained from the BF and AR sites had some measurements lower than the detection limit. In this study, these values were replaced with the values of the detection limit, thus potentially overestimating the actual OMP concentrations.

PCA is a multivariate statistical analysis for determining the key variables in a large set of data. PCA simplifies the analysis and visualization of multidimensional data sets and reveals important variables that are difficult to discover (Raychaudhuri et al., 2000). The BF and AR sites are characterized by a large number of chemical and physical variables; thus, PCA was carried out to reduce a large set of original variables collected in this study and to find factors (principal components, PCs) for representing correlations of many variables (e.g., dissolved oxygen (O_2), residence time, well distance, redox potential, etc.). PCs determined in this study illustrated interrelationships among many original variables with OMP removal at BF and AR sites. PCA was applied using SPSS 16.0 (SPSS Inc, Chicago, Illinois, USA). Table 6.1 shows a list of analyzed parameters used for PCA, the limit of quantification (LOQ), the percent of data below LOQ, and their average concentrations from Lake Tegel (BF) and the recharge pond (AR).

Table 6.1 Summary of analyzed parameters and average concentrations at the BF site and the AR site

Parameters	Unit	LOQ	BF[2] (Average)	MIN	MAX	% <LOQ	AR[3] (Average)	MIN	MAX	% <LOQ
Total organic carbon	mg/L	0.5	7.7	6.1	9.5	0	7.6	6.1	8.8	0
Dissolved organic carbon	mg/L	0.5	7.0	4.7	8.2	0	7.2	6.1	9.6	0
Dissolved oxygen	mg/L	N.A.[1]	11.2	7.2	17.0	N.A.	11.0	6.1	17.6	N.A.[1]
UV254nm	1/m	N.A.[1]	15.7	137	20.9	N.A.	15.6	6.4	19.8	N.A.[1]
pH		N.A.[1]	8.00	7.4	8.5	N.A.	8.06	7.5	9.1	N.A.[1]
Temperature	°C	N.A.[1]	11.2	1.0	24.2	N.A.	11.3	0.2	24.7	N.A.[1]
Oxidation-reduction potential	mV	N.A.[1]	377	291	508	N.A.	372	230	495	N.A.[1]
Ammonia	mg/L	0.04	0.08	0.04	0.25	46	0.08	0.04	0.20	46
Nitrate	mg/L	0.05	1.8	0.48	3.20	0	1.5	0.36	2.40	0
Iron	mg/L	0.03	0.03	0.03	0.03	100	0.04	0.03		67
Manganese	mg/L	0.005	0.02	0.005	0.077	42	0.02	0.005	0.06	37
Calcium	mg/L	0.1	88.4	79.5	102	0	86.7	74.2	100	0
Bicarbonate	mg/L	1.0	177.6	156	207	0	174.0	145	200	0
Sulfate	mg/L	1.0	125.2	92	147	0	120.9	94	142	0
Carbamazepine	µg/L	0.05	0.46	0.14	0.86	0	0.41	0.16	0.93	0
Phenazone	µg/L	0.05	0.34	0.08	0.79	0	0.32	0.12	0.57	0
Propyphenazone	µg/L	0.05	0.06	0.05	0.12	50	0.08	-	-	-
AMDOPH	µg/L	0.05	0.21	0.12	0.29	0	0.14	0.05	0.33	59
1-acetyl-1-methyl-2-phenylhydrazide (AMPH)	µg/L	0.05	0.05	0.05	0.05	100	0.15	0.05	0.28	44
MTBE	µg/L	0.03	0.17	0.03	0.42	4	0.19	0.03	0.49	5

[1]N.A.: Not Applied; [2] BF: bank filtration site; [3] AR: artificial recharge site

6.3. Results and discussion

6.3.1. Temperature

Water temperature plays an important role in the performance of BF and AR and is also often used as a tracer to estimate travel times. Temperature affects bacterial production and abundance, and biodegradation is an important mechanism in removing bulk organic matter during BF and AR (Miettinen et al., 1996; Maeng et al., 2008). Massmann et al. (2006) found that reduced microbial activities from the low temperature of pond water during winter induced more oxic conditions below the AR pond at Lake Tegel. Miettinen et al. (1996) observed that the buffering effect of the ground on temperature for a lake BF site (Lake Kallavesi, Finland) with a short residence time (e.g., 1 week) was weak, resulting in high seasonal variation in microbial activity. Therefore, temperature range variation is an important monitoring parameter for BF and AR systems. In this study the BF and AR sites exhibited different extents of seasonal temperature variation. Maximum temperature variations observed in shallow monitoring wells at the BF site (TEG371OP and TEG372) and the AR site (TEG365 and TEG368OP) were 15°C and 25°C, respectively (Figure 6.4). Maximum temperature variations in deep monitoring wells located at the BF site (3301 and 3302) and the AR site (368UP and 369UP) were 12°C and 20°C, respectively. This was due to the longer residence time (maximum 4.5 months) at the BF site compared to about 50 days at the AR site. Moreover, the shallow monitoring wells (shorter residence times) showed a higher seasonal temperature variation than the deep monitoring wells (longer residence times) at both sites.

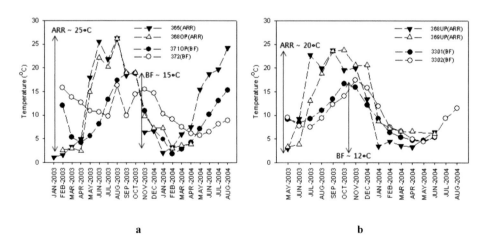

a   b

Figure 6.4 Seasonal temperature variations for BF site and AR sites in Berlin, Germany; (a) two shallow observation wells, (b) two deep observation wells, respectively

6.3.2. Redox conditions

Process sustainability in natural treatment systems (e.g., BF and AR) requires biodegradation to be the most important and dominant removal mechanism (Schmidt et al., 2007). Redox conditions play an important role in biodegradation during BF and AR because they can promote or retard the removal of natural and synthetic organic compounds sensitive to different hydrogeochemical environments (Hiscock and Grischek, 2002). Typically, oxidation-reduction potential (ORP) values above +200 mV correspond to aerobic or oxic conditions where microorganisms use oxygen as a terminal electron acceptor (TEA) during respiration. Anoxic conditions are present between -200 and +200 mV (TEAs: NO_3^-, Mn^{4+}, Fe^{3+} and SO_4^{2-}), and ORP values below -200 mV correspond to anaerobic conditions (TEA: CO_2) (Cronk and Fennessy, 2001; Inniss, 2005). Figure 6.5 illustrates the range of ORP values with respect to travel distances, residence times and depths for BF and AR sites, respectively. ORPs at all monitoring wells showed inverse correlations with respect to travel distances ($R^2 = 0.74$), residence times ($R^2 = 0.73$) and depths ($R^2 = 0.79$) at the BF site (Figure 6.5a, 6.5c and 6.5e). This implies that the BF site shows an oxic zone followed by an anoxic zone which occurs in the deeper wells (> 15 m). In contrast, both shallow and deep monitoring wells at the AR site had higher ORPs associated with mainly oxic conditions regardless of travel distances, residence times and depths. An AR system usually has an unsaturated zone and as a result of the drying period of the wet/dry cycle, re-oxygenation occurs. The AR site had relatively low variations in redox conditions (Figure 6.5b, 6.5d and 6.5f).

Residence times and travel distances showed good inverse correlations with ORP for BF. This implies that residence times and travel distances could be used as an indicator to monitor ORP. However, the correlations observed in this study cannot be applied to other BF sites because the ORP variations are site–specific. Table 6.2 summarizes differences in residence times, redox conditions and temperatures between the Lake Tegel BF site and the AR site.

Table 6.2: Summary of site conditions at field sites

Parameter	BF site	AR site
Residence time	Longer (4.5 months)	Shorter (50 days)
Infiltrate mixing	High incidences of old and young infiltrate mixing resulting in elevated concentrations of certain persistent compounds in the production well	Young infiltrate encountered in wells close to recharge pond and some groundwater impact in production wells
Redox conditions	Short oxic zone followed by a more reduced zone (400 mV to 93 mV)	Mainly oxic zone (387 mV to 309 mV)
Temperature change (season)	Lower (12 – 15°C)	Higher (20 - 25°C)
Temperature influence	Less influence of temperature on redox conditions	Higher influence of temperature leading to seasonal changes in redox conditions

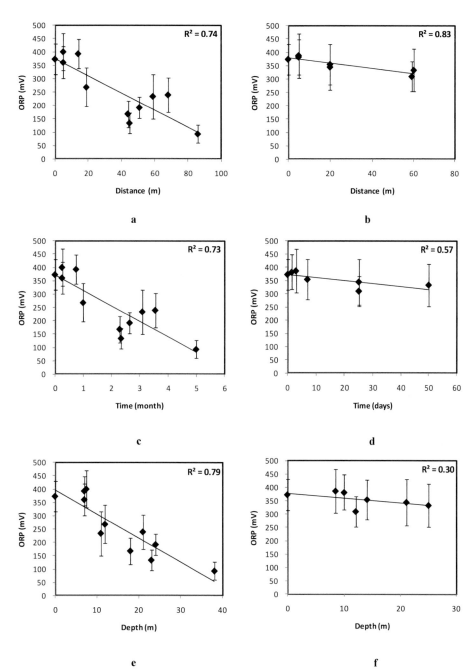

Figure 6.5 Comparison of oxidation-reduction potentials (ORP) with respect to travel distance, residence time and depth between BF (a, c, and e) and AR (b, d, and f) sites (BF: n=8-28, AR: n=7-26)

6.3.3. Organic micropollutants attenuated under oxic conditions

High concentrations of phenazone were observed in the groundwater monitoring well (TEG373: 1.47 ± 0.58 µg/L) at the AR site and the deep monitoring well (TEG374: 1.61 ± 0.33 µg/L) at the BF site. Phenazone input concentrations from Lake Tegel (BF) and the recharge pond (AR) were 0.34 ± 0.10 µg/L and 0.32 ± 0.09 µg/L, respectively (Table 6.1). The share of phenazone-contaminated groundwater in the production well reported by Grünheid et al. (2005) at the AR site was 20%, and this was higher than the share of "old" bank filtrate (7%) which was the only source for phenazone contamination in the production well at the BF site (i.e., no groundwater contamination by phenazone at the BF site) (Figure 6.6). In contrast, the concentration of phenazone at the production well (0.26 ± 0.15 µg/L) at the AR site was relatively low compared to the BF site (0.50 ± 0.14 µg/L). This may due to the predominantly oxic conditions at the AR site which enhance the degradation of phenazone in groundwater as it moves towards the production well.

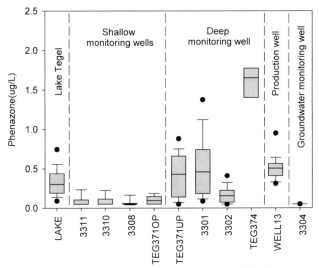

Figure 6.6 Phenazone concentrations along the transect at BF site (no mixing correction, n=14 - 28)

Previous studies have shown that the removal of phenazone-type pharmaceuticals occurs as a result of biodegradation, most of which occurs in the first few meters of the infiltration zone (Massmann et al., 2006; Zuehlke et al., 2007). Phenazone was reported as a redox-sensitive compound that was efficiently biodegraded under oxic conditions (66%) and showed very low removal (10%) under anoxic conditions at the Lake Wannsee field site in Berlin, Germany (Massmann et al., 2008). In addition, FAA (formylaminoantipyrine) and AAA (acetoaminoantipyrine), transformation products from a phenazone-type pharmaceutical (dimethylaminophenazone (DMAA)), were higher at the deep monitoring well TEG374 (ORP: 93 mV, FAA: 0.39 µg/L, AAA: 0.23 µg/L) compared to the shallow monitoring well TEG371OP (ORP: 268 mV, FAA < 0.05

µg/L, AAA < 0.05 µg/L) at the BF site. Being a phenazone-type compound (i.e., transformation product), the removal mechanism for these transformation products is suggested to be the same as that of phenazone (biological transformation) and they appear to be degraded more favorably under oxic conditions. Zuehlke et al. (2007) have detected transformation products of 1,5-dimethyl-1,2-dehydro-3-pyrazolone (DP) and 4-(2-methylethyl)-1,5-dimethyl-1,2-dehydro-3-pyrazolone (PDP) as a result of the biodegradation of phenazone and propyphenazone, respectively. In addition, AMDOPH, another DMAA metabolite, was elevated in monitoring well TEG374 (5.8 µg/L) and the production well (0.83 µg/L) at the BF site (Figure 6.7a).

The mean concentration of phenazone in the production well at the BF site was even higher (0.77 µg/L) after correcting for mixing with ambient groundwater which contains phenazone below the detection limit (0.05 µg/L). The high concentrations of phenazone in the old bank filtrate clearly contributed to the elevated concentrations of phenazone observed. Thus, it was necessary to correct for mixing with old bank filtrate to estimate the reduction of phenazone over a travel (residence) time of 4.5-months. AMDOPH was used as a conservative tracer to estimate the proportion of old bank filtrate in the production well at the BF site because of its persistence in the environment. Previous studies reported that AMDOPH also showed a persistent behavior during conventional drinking water treatment, BF, AR, and laboratory-scale experiments (Reddersen et al., 2002; Massmann et al., 2006; Zuehlke et al., 2007; Massmann et al., 2008). Table 6.3 shows a list of phenazone-type pharmaceuticals and their transformation products with an indicator of biodegradability and octanol-water partition coefficients (log K_{ow}). All residues of phenazone-type pharmaceuticals in Table 6.3 were predicted as being not readily biodegradable compounds using BIOWIN3 and BIOWIN5, as indicated by Estimation Program Interface (EPI) Suite (US EPA, 2009). BIOWIN3 estimates the time required for ultimate biodegradation of an organic compound, and BIOWIN5 assesses the biodegradation probability of an organic compound according to the Japanese MITI (Ministry of International Trade and Industry) ready biodegradation test (US EPA, 2009). A biodegradation probability of greater than 0.5 corresponds to the compound biodegrading fast. When the BIOWIN3 predicts "weeks" or faster (i.e., days or days to weeks) and the BIOWIN5 assesses the probability is greater or equal to 0.5, then the result is YES (readily biodegradable). In contrast, if the prediction is less than 0.5, the prediction is NO (not readily biodegradable). KOWWIN^{TM} was used to estimate log K_{ow} (US EPA, 2009). AMDOPH exhibited the lowest log K_{ow} value and was the most polar/mobile compound among the residues of phenazone-type pharmaceuticals. Thus, this explains why AMDOPH showed a persistent behavior at the BF and AR sites.

Figure 6.7 shows that calculated AMDOPH concentrations changed during adjustment for ambient groundwater (Figure 6.7b) and ambient groundwater with old bank filtrate (Figure 6.7c). Using AMDOPH as a conservative tracer, the proportions of water in the production well were 35%, 7% and 58% for groundwater, old bank filtrate and young bank filtrate, respectively. Pekdeger (2006) suggested the proportions of water in the production well from the BF site at Lake Tegel were 31-42%, 11% and 47-58% for young bank filtrate, old bank filtrate and groundwater, respectively, using a multi-tracer approach. Thus, the proportions for young bank filtrate and groundwater estimated using AMDOPH in this study were in the range of the proportions proposed by Pekdeger (2006). After correcting for mixing with old bank filtrate (TEG374) and deep monitoring wells (TEG371UP, 3301, 3302 and 3303), the phenazone concentrations in the production well No.13 were adjusted from 0.50 µg/L to 0.2 µg/L, and became close to phenazone concentrations exhibited at the shallow monitoring wells at the BF site.

Table 6.3 Biodegradability and log K_{ow} of phenazone-type compounds and metabolites

Name	CAS	MW	Readily biodegradable[a]	log K_{ow}[b]
Phenazone	60-80-0	188.23	NO	0.59
Propyphenazone	479-92-5	230.31	NO	2.05
DMAA (Dimethylaminophenazone)	58-15-1	231.30	NO	0.60
AMDOPH (1-acetyl-1-methyl-2-dimethyloxamoyl-2-phenylhydrazide)	519-65-3	263.30	NO	-0.045
AMPH (1-acetyl-1-methyl-2-phenylhydrazide)	38604-70-5	164.21	NO	1.603
FAA (Formylaminoantipyrine)	1672-5-8-8	231.26	NO	0.882
AAA (Acetoaminoantipyrine)	83-15-8	245.28	NO	0.759
DP (1,5-dimethyl-1,2-dehydro-3-pyrazolone)		112.13	NO	
PDP (4-(2-methylethyl)-1,5-dimethyl-1,2-dehydro-3-pyrazolone)		154.21	NO	

[a] BIOWIN v.4.10 (US EPA, 2009); [b] log K_{ow} estimated by KOWWIN™ (US EPA, 2009)

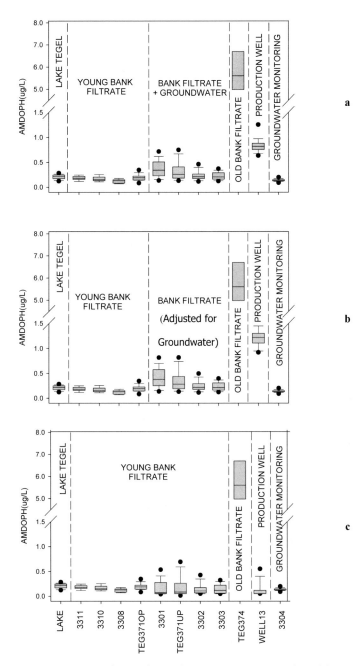

Figure 6.7 AMDOPH concentrations along the transect at BF site: (a) no mixing correction, (b) groundwater correction and (c) groundwater and old bank filtrate correction (n=14-28)

6.3.4. Organic micropollutants attenuated under anoxic conditions

The removals of X-ray contrast agents measured as absorbable organic iodine (AOI) and ORP levels were measured in monitoring wells at the BF site and the AR site. AOI concentrations at the BF site, which exhibits shorter oxic conditions followed by prolonged anoxic conditions, showed a positive correlation ($R^2 = 0.94$) with ORP which implies that AOI reduction was more effective under reducing conditions. In contrast, AOI concentrations were not significantly changed during soil passage at the AR site because of oxic conditions. Therefore, AOI reduction was relatively low compared to the BF site. Jekel and Grünheid (2005) and Grünheid et al. (2005) suggested that AOI reduction observed at the BF site may be attributed to the dehalogenation of AOI which is more likely to occur under reducing conditions. Short residence times and drying periods (promoting oxic conditions) at the AR site may not suitable for degradation of X-ray contrast agents.

Figures 6.8a and 6.8b show the ranges of carbamazepine concentrations along each transect toward the last monitoring well before the production wells at the BF and AR sites, respectively. Mixing corrections for native groundwater and old bank filtrate were taken into account in the estimation of carbamazepine removal efficiency, and the mean concentration of carbamazepine from a native groundwater monitoring well (3304) and old bank filtrate (TEG374) was below the quantification limit (0.05 µg/L). A slight reduction of carbamazepine was observed at the monitoring well 3311 located within the first few meters from Lake Tegel (residence time < 1 month, Grünheid et al. (2005)), while further attenuation occurs along the flow path to the production well 13 reaching a mean removal of 89%. At the AR site, the mean removal of carbamazepine was 35%. A higher concentration of carbamazepine was detected in the production well No. 20 at the AR site compared to the production well 13 at the BF site. As mentioned previously, the BF site had a longer residence time under reducing conditions compared to the AR site, and this may have enhanced the attenuation of carbamazepine. Zhang et al. (2008) summarized previous studies on occurrence and fate of carbamazepine in wastewater treatment processes and water bodies and suggested removal efficiencies were mostly less than 10% during biological wastewater treatment processes because carbamazepine exhibits resistance to biodegradation. In contrast, three wastewater treatment plants located in the UK showed the carbamazepine removal efficiency ranging from 43 to 54% (Zhou et al., 2009). Our investigations showed that carbamazepine was attenuated about 89% during BF. Elevated carbamazepine concentrations had been observed in Lake Tegel from October 2002 until November 2003, and this (lagged) trend through the transect would have shown if carbamazepine was persistent. However, according to Scheytt et al. (2006), the retardation factor of carbamazepine was 1.84, based on laboratory-scale sand column transport experiments. Carbamazepine concentrations would have appeared in the production about a year later if a retardation factor of 2 was assumed, but no samples from the production well or monitoring wells in its vicinity showed elevated concentration of carbamazepine. More long-term data may be needed to confirm the removal of carbamazepine observed at the BF site.

The removals of X-ray contrast agents measured as AOI, and carbamazepine appear to be generally higher at the BF site than at the AR site.

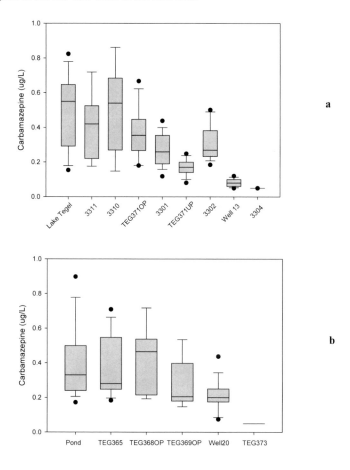

Figure 6.8 Carbamazepine concentrations at (a) BF site and (b) AR site (corrected for mixing) (BF site: n=13-28, AR site: n=8-27)

6.3.5. Principal component analysis – Bank filtration site

Data used for PCA were not corrected for groundwater and old bank filtrate because the PCA is used to explain hydrogeochemical conditions with OMPs using 22 original variables from the BF site and the AR site during the time of the study (with mixing as one possible factor). Moreover, there are a number of variables which could not be accurately corrected for groundwater and old bank filtrate (e.g., redox potential and pH). In this study, loading plots were used to depict a group of original variables based on each PC, and score plots were used to show the projection of original data onto new space, determined by the loadings (Felipe-Sotelo et al., 2008).

For the BF site the PCA revealed the presence of five principal components (PCs) which explained a total variance of 77%. The selected number of components was based on Kaiser's criterion that only components with eigenvalues of 1.0 or more are retained. Five PCs, with eigenvalues exceeding 1, explained 37%, 18%, 11%, 6% and 5% of the variance, respectively. The most significant PCs are the first PC (PC1), which explains 37% of data variability, and the second PC (PC2), which had an explained variance of 18%. The remaining PCs with less explained variance did not reveal additional information about the BF site.

As shown in Figure 6.9b, PC1 (37% explained variance) embodies redox-sensitive parameters with high positive (iron, ammonia, and manganese) and high negative (ORP, O_2 (dissolved oxygen), and nitrate) loadings. Depth, residence time and well distance (positive loadings on PC1) are clearly grouped and correlated with concentrations of iron, manganese and ammonia (positive loadings on PC1) and inversely correlated with ORP and O_2 (negative loadings on PC1). As shown earlier (Figure 6.5), redox conditions became more reduced as depth, travel time and distance increased. The compounds located in the upper-left quadrant (high negative loadings on PC1) are stable under oxic condition (e.g., nitrate and carbamazepine). Moreover, PC1 gave high positive loadings for transformation products of phenazone-type pharmaceuticals (e.g., AMDOPH and AMPH (1-acetyl-1-methyl-2-phenylhydrazide)) because these compounds were formed by oxic biotransformation and remained stable under anoxic conditions.

PC2 explained 18% of the total variance. Total organic carbon (TOC) and dissolved organic carbon (DOC) showed strong positive loadings, while time, distance, depth, HCO_3^-, alkalinity and Ca^{2+} showed strong negative loadings. Thus, PC2 embodied the degradation of organic matter (i.e., degradation potential) and apparently calcium carbonate dissolution potential. The removal efficiency of organic matter during bank filtration increases with residence times and travel distances. This is generally true for most of bank filtration sites where organic matter concentrations are inversely correlated with residence times and travel distances (Lenk et al., 2005). PC2 can be also defined as the calcium carbonate dissolution potential because of its high negative loadings for Ca^{2+}, and HCO_3^-. This suggests that calcium carbonate dissolution occurred during soil passage and gradually increased along the flow path. Dissolved CO_2 released from respiration or oxidation of organic matter by microorganisms in a biological active layer reacts with water to form carbonic acid (H_2CO_3) which reacts with calcium carbonate in the sediment to form bicarbonate (HCO_3^-) according to the following reaction:

$$CaCO_3 + CO_2(g) + H_2O \rightarrow Ca^{2+} + 2HCO_3^- \qquad (2)$$

The score plot of PC1 versus PC2 shows that samples were clustered in different groups based on their (well) sampling locations (Figure 6.9c). Samples shown on the right section of the plot (high positive scores of PC1) are associated with more reducing conditions (deep monitoring wells and production well). In contrast, samples on the left section of the score plot correspond to more oxic conditions (shallow monitoring wells and Lake Tegel). The variation in degradation potential (PC2) was relatively wide between Lake Tegel (the source) and the shallow monitoring wells characterized by aerobic biodegradation. This leads to the conclusion that a biologically active layer under oxic conditions in the shallow parts of the aquifer plays an important role in the degradation of organic matter in a BF system.

The arrows between Lake Tegel and the production well in Figure 6.9a represent the flow paths at the BF site (modified from Massmann et al. (2006) and Pekdeger (2006)). The general flow path can also be derived from the loading and score plots of PC1 and PC2. In Figure 6.9b, variables that showed high negative loadings in PC1 and high positive loadings in PC2 (i.e., the upper-left quadrant of the loading plot) are correlated with the lake (source). On the other hand, variables closely associated with the production well are located at the lower-right quadrant of the loading plot, and characterized by anoxic conditions (PC1) with low degradation potential/calcium carbonate dissolution potential (PC2). As mentioned before, the BF site exhibited oxic conditions followed by reducing conditions; thus the flow path begins from the upper-left quadrant of the loading plot followed by the lower-left quadrant (i.e., calcium carbonate dissolution) and the lower-right quadrant of the loading plot. In fact, Figure 6.9c shows that the general flow path was drawn from samples clustered for the lake (source) followed by the groups of shallow monitoring wells, deep monitoring wells and the production well, and the flow path was similar to the path indicated in the loading plot (Figure 6.9b).

142

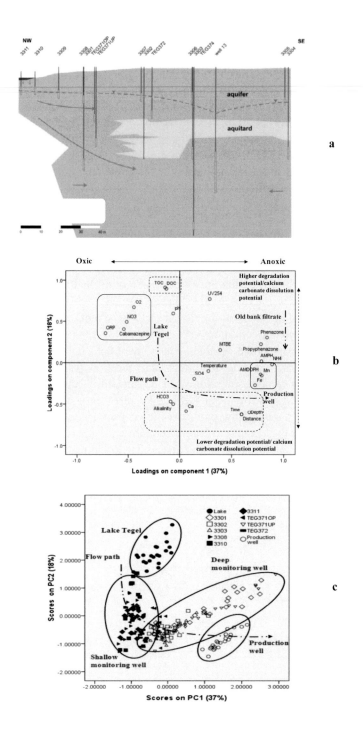

Figure 6.9 PCA of BF data: (a) cross-section of BF site transect showing the flow paths, (b) representation of PC1 versus PC2 loadings, (c) plots of PC1 versus PC2 scores

6.3.6. Principal component analysis – Artificial recharge site

The PCA for the AR site revealed the presence of five components with eigenvalues exceeding 1, explaining 38%, 18%, 14%, 8% and 6% of the variance, respectively, thus explaining a total variance of 84%. PC1 represents redox related parameters like O_2, ORP, Mn and Fe, and explained 38% of total variance, similar to the BF site. PC2 explained 18% of the total variance, and appears to reflect seasonal variation (i.e., temperature variation) with variation of TOC and DOC concentrations. The remaining components; PC3, PC4, and PC5; did not reveal additional information about the AR site. Figure 6.10b shows that temperature exhibits moderate negative loadings on PC2 with time and distance. TOC, DOC and O_2 showed high positive loadings on PC2. Generally, high temperatures during summer enhance microbial activity which reduces DOC and O_2 concentrations. Thus, high temperatures were inversely correlated with concentrations of DOC and O_2. This corresponds to the initial interpretation of the data by Massmann et al. (2006). The score plot (Figure 6.10c) showed that the variations in PC2 for the recharge pond and shallow monitoring wells were relatively higher than that of the deep monitoring wells. The seasonal temperature variations were greater in shallow monitoring wells and the recharge pond.

The elevated phenazone concentrations in groundwater at the AR site gave high positive loadings on PC1. Phenazone would have appeared in the upper-left quadrant of the loading plots (negative loadings on PC1) if it originated from the recharge pond. Transformation products of phenazone-type pharmaceuticals (e.g., AMDOPH and AMPH) are formed during oxic biotransformation and remained stable under anoxic conditions (moderately positive loadings on PC1). On the other hand, carbamazepine is located in the lower-left quadrant of the loading plot. The mean concentration of carbamazepine from a native groundwater monitoring well (TEG373) was below the quantification limit (0.05 µg/L) (Figure 6.8b); thus, carbamazepine was mainly introduced into the AR site from the recharge pond (i.e., oxic conditions which reflect high negative loadings on PC1) and showed low degradation potential (i.e., moderate negative loadings on PC2).

Figure 6.10a presents the flow paths at the AR site. Figures 6.10b and 6.10c also show the general flow paths in the loading plots and the score plots using PC1 and PC2, respectively. In Figure 6.10b, variables having high negative loadings on PC1 and high positive loadings on PC2 (i.e., the upper-left quadrant of loading plots) exhibit high values in the recharge pond (i.e., they represent oxic conditions with a high degradation potential). On the other hand, variables associated with the production well are located in the lower-right quadrant of loading plots and are characterized by anoxic conditions (PC1) with low degradation potential (PC2). Moreover, Figure 6.10c shows the general flow path in the score plot. The flow path starts from samples clustered for the recharge pond followed by the groups of shallow monitoring wells, deep monitoring wells and the production well. As shown in Figure 6.7c, more samples were associated with oxic conditions compared to anoxic conditions.

144

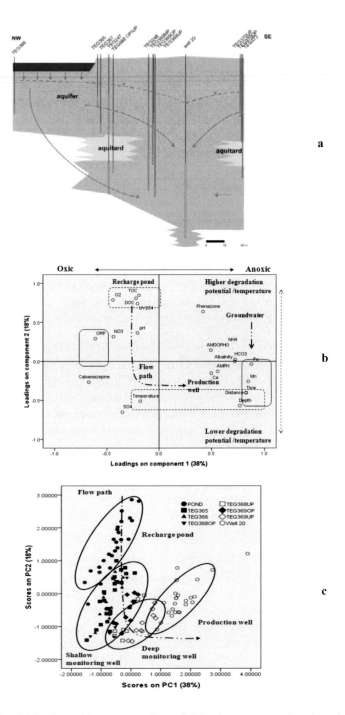

Figure 6.10 PCA of AR data: (a) cross-section of AR site transect showing the flow paths, (b) representation of PC1 versus PC2 loadings, (c) plots of PC1 versus PC2 scores

6.4. Conclusions

Data from the NASRI project were compiled and analyzed in order to investigate factors that influenced OMP removals. Out of the many factors that can influence the performance of soil/aquifer-based natural treatment systems for OMP removals, redox conditions were identified as of major importance. Redox conditions observed at the BF site were oxic in the first few meters followed by reducing conditions (i.e., anoxic conditions). On the other hand, the AR site showed oxic conditions throughout the subsurface passage from the recharge pond to the production well. This study confirms that it is necessary to account for not only mixing from ambient groundwater but also the possible mixing with old bank filtrate while estimating the performance of a BF system – especially under conditions with strong vertical stratification as encountered in Berlin, Germany.

Seasonal temperature variations gave a first indication of differences between the two investigated sites: at the BF site shallow and deep monitoring wells showed maximum variations of 15°C and 12°C, respectively. In contrast, the maximum temperature variations observed at the shallow monitoring wells and the deep monitoring wells at the AR site were 25°C and 20°C, respectively. Thus, the BF site had less temperature variation than the AR site, and this may due to a longer residence time and a higher share of mixing with "old" bank filtrate at the BF site. For OMP removal, phenazone-type pharmaceuticals including phenazone, propyphenazone and the transformation products FAA and AAA were found to be redox-dependent compounds which showed better removal under oxic conditions; thus, they were removed to a higher degree at the AR site. On the other hand, the transformation product AMDOPH was not eliminated either at the BF site or at the AR site. X-ray contrast agents measured as AOI were removed to a greater degree at the BF site. Carbamazepine also showed a higher removal at the BF site compared to that at the AR site. PCA revealed two PCs that were mainly comprised of variables embodying redox conditions (PC1) and degradation potential/calcium carbonate dissolution potential (PC2) at the BF site. At the AR site, redox conditions and temperature with degradation potential were embodied by PC1 and PC2, respectively. The results extracted from the PCA help to understand OMP removals under different hydrogeochemical conditions. PCA indicated that redox conditions play an important role in understanding OMP removals and parameters that influence the performance of BF and AR. PCA analysis is a useful tool to investigate inter-correlations among many variables observed at the BF and AR sites and illustrates the dependence between OMPs and hydrogeochemical conditions. Our understanding of OMP removal in BF and AR systems can be improved using a multivariate analysis (PCA) which was well-suited in this study due to the large amounts of available data.

The degree of risk associated with pharmaceutical residues selected in this study to the environment and public health is not known yet. Therefore, the presence of some pharmaceutical contamination in monitoring wells observed in this study should not be used as a basis for risk assessment in drinking water. A long-term study is still needed to assuredly determine the fate of the residues during soil passage due to long residence times during BF and AR systems.

6.5. References

Cloutier, V., Lefebvre, R., Therrien, R. and Savard, M.M., 2008. Multivariate statistical analysis of geochemical data as indicative of the hydrogeochemical evolution of groundwater in a sedimentary rock aquifer system. J. Hydrol. 353 (3-4), 294-313.

Cronk, J.K. and Fennessy, M.S., 2001. Wetland Plants: Biology and Ecology CRC Press.

Cunningham, V.L., Bunzy, M., Hutchinson, T., Mastrocco, F., Parke, N. and Roden, N., 2006. Effects of human pharmaceuticals on aquatic life: next step. Environ. Sci. Technol. 40 (11), 3456-3462.

Davis, J.C., 1986. Statistics and Data Analysis in Geology. John Wiley & Sons Inc., New York.

Eckert, P. and Irmscher, R., 2006. Over 130 years of experience with Riverbank Filtration in Düsseldorf, Germany. J. Water Supply Res. T. 55 (4), 283-291.

Felipe-Sotelo, M., Tauler, R., Vives, I. and Grimalt, J.O., 2008. Assessment of the environmental and physiological processes determining the accumulation of organochlorine compounds in European mountain lake fish through multivariate analysis (PCA and PLS). Sci. Total Environ. 404 (1), 148-161.

Fritz, B., 2003. Introduction. NASRI Workshop 2003. Berlin Centre of Competence for Water (KWB), Berlin.

Greskowiak, J., Prommer, H., Massmann, G., Nützmann, G. and Pekdeger, A., 2005. The impact of variably saturated conditions on hydrogeochemical changes during artificial recharge of groundwater. Applied Geochemistry, 20 (7), 1409-1426.

Grünheid, S., Amy, G. and Jekel, M., 2005. Removal of bulk dissolved organic carbon (DOC) and trace organic compounds by bank filtration and artificial recharge. Water Res. 39 (14), 3219.

Halling-Soensen, B., Nors Nielsen, S., Lanzky, P.F., Ingerslev, F., Holten Luzhot, H.C. and Jogensen, S.E., 1998. Occurrence, fate and effects of pharmaceutical substances in the environment- A review. Chemosphere 36 (2), 357-393.

Heberer, T., 2002a. Occurrence, fate, and removal of pharmaceutical residues in the aquatic environment: a review of recent research data. Toxicol. Lett. 131, 5-17.

Heberer, T., 2002b. Tracking persistent pharmaceutical residues from municipal sewage to drinking water. J. Hydrol. 266 (3-4), 175-189.

Heberer, T., Mechlinski, A., Fanck, B., Knappe, A., Massmann, G., Pekdeger, A. and Fritz, B., 2004. Field Studies on the Fate and Transport of Pharmaceutical Residues in Bank Filtration. Ground Water Monit. R. 24 (2), 70-77.

Hiscock, K.M. and Grischek, T., 2002. Attenuation of groundwater pollution by bank filtration. J. Hydrol. 266 (3-4), 139-144.

Inniss, E.C. (Ed.), 2005. Use of Redox Potentials in Wastewater Treatment. Wiley Interscience.

Irmscher, R. and Teermann, I., 2002. Riverbank filtration for drinking water supply - a proven method, perfect to face today's challenge. Water Sci. Technol. 2 (5-6), 1-8.

Jekel, M. and Grünheid, S., 2005. Bank filtration and groundwater recharge for treatment of polluted surface waters. Water Sci. Technol. 5 (5), 57-66.

Kim, S.D., Cho, J., Kim, I.S., Vanderford, B.J. and Snyder, S.A., 2007. Occurrence and removal of pharmaceuticals and endocrine disruptors in South Korean surface, drinking, and waste waters. Water Res. 41 (5), 1013-1021.

Lenk, S., Remmler, F., Skark, C. and Zullei-Seibert, N., 2005. Removal capacity of riverbank filtration and conclusions for the operation of water abstraction plants. 5th international symposium on management of aquifer recharge, 10-16 June 2005, Berlin, Germany.

Maeng, S.K., Sharma, S.K., Amy, G. and Magic-Knezev, A., 2008. Fate of effluent organic matter (EfOM) and natural organic matter (NOM) through riverbank filtration. Water Sci. Technol. 57 (12), 1999–2007.

Massmann, G., Dunnbier, U., Heberer, T. and Taute, T., 2008. Behaviour and redox sensitivity of pharmaceutical residues during bank filtration - Investigation of residues of phenazone-type analgesics. Chemosphere 71 (8), 1476-1485.

Massmann, G., Greskowiak, J., Dünnbier, U. and Zuehlke, S., 2006. The impact of variable temeratures on the redox conditions and the behavior of pharmaceutical residues during artifical recharge. J. Hydrol. 328, 141-156.

Miettinen, I.T., Vartiainen, T. and Martikainen, P.J., 1996. Bacterial enzyme activities in ground water during bank filtration of lake water. Water Res. 30 (10), 2495-2501.

Pekdeger, A., 2006. Hydrogeological-hydrogeochemical processes during bank filtration and groundwater recharge using a multi tracer approach. NASRI Project, Berlin.

Raychaudhuri, S., Stuart, J.M. and Altman, R.B., 2000. Principal components analysis to summarize microarray experiments: application to sporulation time series. Pacific symposium on biocomputing, Hawaii, USA, 452-463.

Reddersen, K., Heberer, T. and Dünnbier, U., 2002. Identification and significance of phenazone drugs and their metabolites in ground-and drinking water. Chemosphere 49 (6), 539-544.

Scheytt, T.J., Mermann, P. and Heberer, T., 2006. Mobility of pharmaceuticals carbamazepine, diclofenac, ibuprofen, and propyphenazone in miscible-displacement experiments. J. Contam. Hydrol. 83, 53-69.

Schmidt, C.K., Lange, F.T. and Brauch, H.J., 2007. Characteristics and evaluation of natural attenuation processes for organic micropollutant removal during riverbank filtration. Regional IWA conference on Groundwater management in the Danube river basin and other large river basins, Belgrade, 231-236.

Schwab, B.W., 2005. Human pharmaceuticals in U.S. Surface Water: A Human Health Risk Assesment. Regul. Toxicol. Pharm. 42, 296-312.

Snyder, S.A., Leising, J., Westerhoff, P., Yoon, Y., Mash, H. and Vanderford, B., 2004. Biological and Physical Attenuation of Endocrine Disruptors and Pharmaceuticals: Implications for Water Reuse. Ground Water Monit. R. 24 (2), 108-118.

US EPA, 2009. Estimation Programs Interface Suite™ for Microsoft® Windows, v 4.00. United States Environmental Protection Agency, Washington, DC, USA.

Zhang, Y., Geissen, S.-U. and Gal, C., 2008. Carbamazepine and diclofenac: Removal in wastewater treatment plants and occurrence in water bodies. Chemosphere 73 (8), 1151-1161.

Zhou, J.L., Zhang, Z.L., Banks, E., Grover, D. and Jiang, J.Q., 2009. Pharmaceutical residues in wastewater treatment works effluents and their impact on receiving river water. J. Hazard. Mater. 166 (2-3), 655-661.

Zuehlke, S., Duennbier, U. and Heberer, T., 2007. Investigation of the behavior and metabolism of pharmaceutical residues during purification of contaminated ground water used for drinking water supply. Chemosphere 69 (11), 1673-1680.

Chapter 7

FRAMEWORK FOR ASSESSMENT OF ORGANIC MICROPOLLUTANTS REMOVALS DURING MANAGED AQUIFER RECHARGE

Parts of this chapter were based on:

Maeng, S.K., Sharma, S.K., Amy G.L., 2010. Framework for assessment of organic micropollutant (OMP) removals during managed aquifer recharge and recovery (MAR): In "Riverbank filtration for Water Security in Desert Countries", C. Ray and M. Shamrukh (eds), NATO Science for Peace and Security Series, Springer, Dordrecht, The Netherlands, (In Press).

Maeng, S.K. Sharma, S.K. and Amy G.L., 2010. Modelling of removal of wastewater-derived organic micropollutants during managed aquifer recharge and recovery, Water Science and Technology, Accepted.

Summary

Managed aquifer recharge (MAR) is a reliable and proven treatment process, in which water quality can be improved by different physical, biological, and chemical reactions during soil passage. MAR can potentially be included in a multi-barrier treatment system for organic micropollutant (OMP) removal in drinking water treatment and wastewater reuse schemes. However, there is a need to develop assessment tools to help implement MAR as an effective barrier in attenuating different OMPs including pharmaceutically active compounds (PhACs) and endocrine disrupting compounds (EDCs). In this study, guidelines were developed for different classes of OMPs, in which removal efficiencies of these compounds are determined as a function of travel times and distances. Guidelines are incorporated into simple Microsoft Excel spreadsheets and the water quality prediction tool was developed to estimate the removal of different classes of OMPs in MAR systems. Multiple linear regression analysis of data obtained from literature studies showed that travel (residence) time is one of the main parameters in estimating the performance of a MAR system for PhACs removal. Moreover, a quantitative structure activity relationship (QSAR) based model was proposed to predict OMP removals. The QSAR approach is especially useful for emerging compounds with little information about their fate during soil passage. Such an assessment framework for OMP removals is useful for adapting MAR as a multi-objective (-contaminant) barrier and understanding the fate of different classes of compounds during soil passage and the determination of post treatment requirements for MAR.

7.1. Introduction

Managed aquifer recharge (MAR) has been applied in Europe for more than 100 years as a natural water treatment process. MAR is a robust and proven process for water quality improvement, and it can provide a good quality of raw water to water utilities (Ray, 2008). In MAR systems, there are different ways to infiltrate water from sources (e.g., river, lake and infiltration basin) to an aquifer using a hydraulic gradient. First, riverbank filtration (RBF) or lake bank filtration (LBF) uses the hydraulic gradient between the river/lake and a production well (aquifer), and this is an efficient approach where an aquifer is hydraulically connected to the river or lake (Díaz-Cruz and Barceló, 2008). Second, artificial recharge (AR) or soil aquifer treatment (SAT) systems use an infiltration basin to induce water to a recovery well. To introduce water into an infiltration basin, the water has to be pumped from the river or lake (or a wastewater treatment plant in the case of SAT). In this way, AR and SAT systems have relatively fewer impacts from flooding conditions, whereas in RBF the elevated river stage increases the contribution of river to a production well (i.e., less groundwater) (Ray et al., 2002). However, AR systems require more land area for an infiltration basin and may lead to groundwater contamination in the case of persistent contaminants in the source water.

Many studies have been conducted to investigate the fate of wastewater-derived organic micropollutants (OMPs) during MAR and determine the feasibility of MAR as a multi-objective (-contaminant) barrier for OMP removals in indirect potable reuse schemes (Díaz-Cruz and Barceló, 2008; Schmidt et al., 2007; Massmann et al., 2006). However, there are a number of considerations such as design and operational conditions that must be established for the barrier to be effective in attenuating a range of wastewater-derived OMPs including pharmaceutically active compounds (PhACs), endocrine disrupting compounds (EDCs) and personal care products (PCPs) (Hiscock and Grischek, 2002). Depending on the physicochemical properties of OMPs and other water quality parameters, the principal removal mechanism(s) (e.g., sorption and/or biodegradation) during soil passage may vary at different sites (Schmidt et al., 2003).

QSAR (quantitative structure activity relationship), also referred to as quantitative structure-property relationships (QSPR), have long been used in the pharmaceutical industry to predict the metabolic activity of drugs as a function of compound physicochemical properties. QSAR models have been developed and used in environmental sciences to estimate the toxicity of pollutants as a function of their physicochemical properties (Tao et al., 2002). There has been recent interest in further application of QSAR approaches to predicting water treatment performance in removing OMPs as a function of compound physicochemical properties. Emerging OMPs, including EDCs, PhAC, and PCPs, represent a major concern in drinking water treatment and wastewater reclamation/reuse. A QSAR approach links compound properties (i.e., structure) to the removals (activity). Furthermore, it is important to have reliable datasets in order to develop a QSAR model because there are many factors that can influence the removal of OMPs during soil passage. Therefore, in this chapter, input data used for QSAR model development were obtained from soil column studies that were conducted using identical experimental set-ups with a single protocol for PhACs measurements (Chapter 5). Moreover, these laboratory-scale soil column studies were conducted to investigate the role of biodegradation in OMP removals during MAR.

The prediction of OMP removals during soil passage is important in case of an unintentional release of OMPs into drinking water sources (e.g., river and lake). This is a major concern for water utilities to prepare post treatment requirements to eliminate OMPs in drinking water. In this study, guidelines were proposed to estimate removal efficiencies of OMPs and a prediction tool based on databases was developed to aid in the design of a MAR system. Moreover, a QSAR model was used to estimate the removal of OMPs during soil passage and is especially useful for those OMPs with limited information (i.e., new chemicals).

7.2. Methods for guideline and model development

Figure 7.1 shows a diagram of different steps in the development of a framework for OMP removal by MAR.

7.2.1. Guidelines for estimating removal efficiencies of OMPs

Guidelines for assessment of OMP removal in MAR systems are based on a literature survey and include removal efficiencies of OMPs from MAR field sites. Table 2.3 in Chapter 2 shows summary of field sites that are used for guidelines development. The guidelines enable users to estimate the removal efficiencies based on either a known travel time or travel distance from a water source (e.g., lake or river).

7.2.2. Dataset for QSAR model development

First, 282 cases of PhACs removal efficiencies were used from literature studies. These data are from different MAR sites: 178 corresponding to LBF, 73 RBF and 31 AR. All datasets of OMPs collected from the MAR sites are heterogeneous because of different hydrogeological and hydrogeochemical conditions. The most significant parameters which influence the removal of OMP during soil passage was determined using a multiple linear regression

(MLR) analysis.

One of the limiting factors in the development of a QSAR model for MAR is the quality of experimental data (Walker et al., 2003). Therefore, input data from soil column studies (Chapter 5) conducted using identical experimental set-ups with a single protocol for PhACs measurements were used to develop QSAR models. The experimental data of 13 selected pharmaceuticals were collected from laboratory-scale studies, simulating a bank filtration system and used as a training set to develop the QSAR model to investigate the influence of physicochemical properties of selected PhACs. The data comprised 65 cases of 13 selected PhACs studied in soil column simulations, and their removal efficiencies were designated as dependent variables. A detailed description of materials and methods used for the experimental set-ups is elaborated in Chapter 5.

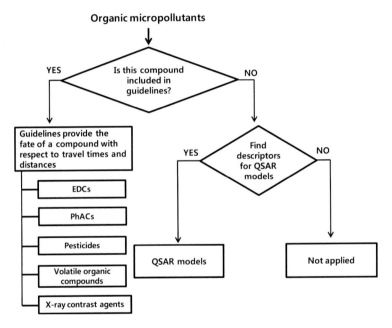

Figure 7.1 Diagram of processing steps in the development and application of framework for assessment of organic micropollutant removal during MAR

7.2.3. Molecular descriptors

Different types of molecular descriptors were calculated and used in this study: constitutional descriptors, connectivity indices and functional groups. 247 descriptors calculated from software packages including DRAGON (Talete, 2009), EPI suite (US EPA, 2009) and Chem3D (Cambridge, 2002) were used to develop QSAR models. For example, connectivity indices, functional groups and constitutional descriptors were calculated from DRAGON. Octanol/water partition coefficients (K_{ow}) were computed using EPI suite, and model outputs from BIOWIN 1-7 were also used. Quantum-chemical descriptors such as highest occupied molecular orbital (HOMO), lowest unoccupied molecular orbital (LUMO) and heat of formation were calculated by a semi-empiric method MOPAC-PM3 (optimization geometry of a molecule) (Yangali-Quintanilla et al., 2010). Operational parameters such as travel distances and travel times were initially considered for inclusion to define parameters that influence the performance of MAR based on literature data. However, operational parameters (e.g., infiltration rate) were excluded for a QSAR model developed based on soil column experiments because the experiment was conducted under the same conditions. Table 7.1 summarizes the types of descriptors used for the model development.

Table 7.1 Types of descriptors used for the development of QSAR model

Descriptor types	Number of descriptors	References
Constitutional descriptors	48	DRAGON[1]
Connectivity indices	33	DRAGON[1]
Functional group counts	154	DRAGON[1]
log K_{ow}, BIOWIN 1-7	8	EPI Suite[2]
Quantum-chemical descriptors	4	Chem3D[3]
Operation parameters	2	

[1] DRAGON 2007 for MS windows, Version 5.5
[2] US EPA 2009 Estimation programs interface suite[TM] for MS windows
[3] Chem3D 2002 Ultra 7.0

7.2.4. Model techniques and validation

A MLR analysis, a common approach to develop a QSAR model, was performed. First, a training set was obtained from literature studies, and 282 cases of PhACs pharmaceutical removal efficiencies were used. These data are from different MAR sites: 178 corresponding to LBF, 73 RBF and 31 AR. MLR analysis was performed using the statistical package SPSS Statistics 16.0. Separate QSAR models were developed for different therapeutic usages classes of OMPs. However, all cases came from different conditions. For example, each site has different hydrogeochemical conditions; hence, it is not possible to come up with a QSAR model which has general applicability. Therefore, a QSAR model was developed based on soil column studies which were carried out in the laboratory to determine descriptors that are important to consider.

A QSAR model should not be used for reproducing known data from training sets, but rather provides more understanding of the behavior of new compounds. Thus, validation is a critical aspect of the QSAR model development for its reliability. Leave-one-out (LOO) cross validation, the most commonly used method for internal validation, was used to estimate the robustness and predictivity of the model (Ghasemi et al., 2009). The goodness of prediction parameter, Q^2 (1-PRESS/TSS, where PRESS is the predictive error sum of squares, and TSS is the total sum of squares), indicates the predictive power of a model (Yangali-Quintanilla et al., 2010). During the LOO cross validation method, a single case from the training set is excluded at a time, and the remaining cases were used as the training data set to predict the single case. This process was repeated until each case in the training set had been used for prediction by developed models. Moreover, an external validation was also carried out to verify the reliability of the model. Validating QSAR models using external data greatly enhances the prediction power of a QSAR model and its applicability. In this study, 26 cases of PhACs (removal efficiency) obtained from literature surveys in Chapter 2 (constituting a heterogeneous data set) were used as external validation data.

7.3. Results and discussion

7.3.1. Guidelines for organic micropollutants removal

An assessment of OMP removals during MAR comprised different groups of OMPs including PhACs, EDCs and pesticides. The ranges of removal efficiencies for different groups of OMPs as a function of travel times and distances were defined using scatter plots with delineation of bins which were then summarized in tables (Table 7.2, 7.3 and 7.4). For example, the scatter plots of EDCs data against travel times and distances at MAR sites were compiled and shown in Figure 7.2. The scatter plots are required to determine the removal ranges of EDCs in the guidelines. According to Figure 7.2, EDCs concentrations were reduced gradually as travel distances and travel times increased. EDCs removal exceeds 65% when MAR sites exhibit greater than 10 meters of travel distances and 10 days of travel times. EDCs are generally known to have high log K_{ow} values (indicating hydrophobicity) and are neutral compounds; thus, adsorption is an important mechanism for the removal of EDCs. PhACs consist of many different compounds, which show different physicochemical properties, with respect to their usages. Two principal removal mechanisms are responsible for the removal of PhACs: adsorption and biodegradation. Therefore, the developed guidelines can be enhanced by classifying their usages; thus, there is one guideline for each type of PhACs (e.g., antibiotics and lipid regulators). Guidelines for MAR systems aid in preliminary assessment of removal of a compound or different classes of compounds. Moreover, Table 7.5, 7.6 and 7.7 show summary of proposed guidelines for PhACs, X-Ray contrast agents and pesticides, respectively.

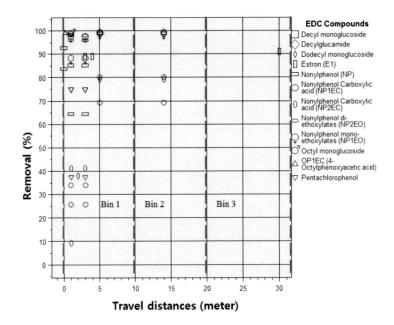

(a)

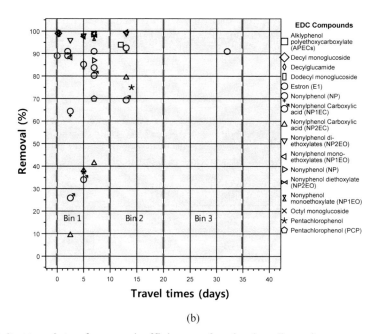

(b)

Figure 7.2 Scatter plots of removal efficiency of endocrine disrupting compounds with (a) travel distances and (b) travel times

Table 7.2 Analysis of scatter plot of endocrine disrupting compound removals with travel distances

Influent (µg/L)	Effluent (µg/L)	Distance (m)	Removal (%)	No. of cases	Average (µg/L)	Standard deviation (µg/L)	Prediction (%)
0.0009 - 1000	0.0001 - 22.4	0-10	9-99	40	75	27	48-74
		10-20	69-100	11	87	13	74 - 91
		20-35	91	1	91		> 91
		Total No.		52			

Table 7.3 Analysis of scatter plot of endocrine disrupting compound removals with travel times

Influent (µg/L)	Effluent (µg/L)	Time (days)	Removal (%)	No. of cases	Average (µg/L)	Standard deviation (µg/L)	Prediction (%)
0.0009 – 1000	0.0001 - 22.4	0-10	9-100	37	72	27	45 - 75
		10-20	69-100	6	88	13	75 - 91
		20-32	91	2	91	-	> 91
		Total No.		45			

Table 7.4 Summary of proposed guidelines for the removal of endocrine disrupting compounds with respect to travel distances and travel times

Influent Range (μg/L)	Effluent Range (μg/L)	Distance (m)	Removal (%)	Travel Time (days)	Removal (%)
0.0009 – 1000	0.01 - 22.4	0-10	48-74	0-10	45 - 75
		10-20	74 - 91	10-20	75 - 91
		20-35	>91	20-32	> 91

Table 7.5 Summary of proposed guidelines for the removal of pharmaceutically active compounds with respect to travel distances and travel times

Influent Range (μg/L)	Effluent Range (μg/L)	Distance (m)	Removal (%)	Travel Time (days)	Removal (%)
0.015 - 520	0.0 - 290	0-20	23-54	0-10	12-45
		20-45	54-58	10-40	45-58
		45-70	58-75	40-60	58-72
		70-85	75-87	60-80	72-80

Table7.6 Summary of proposed guidelines for the removal of X-ray contrast agents with respect to travel distances and travel times

Influent Range (μg/L)	Effluent Range (μg/L)	Distance (m)	Removal (%)	Travel Time (days)	Removal (%)
0.7 – 14.9	0.0 – 10.3	0-28	41-53	0-20	48-56
		28-45	53-77	20-40	56-67
		45-70	77-80	40-75	67-76
		70-85	80-91	75-100	76-80
		85-105	91-100	100-125	80-90
				125-140	90-100

Table 7.7 Summary of proposed guidelines for the removal of pesticides with respect to travel distances and travel times

Influent Range (μg/L)	Effluent Range (μg/L)	Distance (m)	Removal (%)	Travel Time (days)	Removal (%)
0 – 29.35	0 – 22.86	0-20	20 - 38	9 - 90	23 - 67
		20-40	38 - 58	20 - 99	67 - 86
		40-110	58 - 70	30 -86	>86
		110 - 190	70 - 82		
		190 - 230	82 - 99		

7.3.2. Guidelines for removal of different classes of PhACs

Based on the literature review of MAR field sites, scatter plots for 6 different classes of PhACs were prepared to investigate the behavior of different PhACs during soil passage:

Blood lipid regulators

Blood lipid regulators consist of bezafibrate (BEZ), diethylenetriaminepentaacetic acid (DTP), clofibric acid (CLO), fenofibric acid (FEN) and gemfibrozil (GEM), and their fates during soil passage were investigated using previous LBF field studies (Lakes Tegel and Wannsee in Germany) (Heberer and Adam, 2004; Heberer et al., 2003b; Heberer et al., 2004; Pekdeger, 2006; Scheytt et al., 2004; Verstraeten et al., 2002). The generated scatter plots show the removal efficiencies for blood lipid regulators with travel times and travel distances and are presented below in Figure 7.3 and Figure 7.4. The analysis of each of 5 bins created for the removal of blood lipid regulators with travel times and travel distances is summarized in Table 7.8 and Table 7.9, respectively. It can be noted that most of the data points occur above 50%, within travel times of 0 - 200 days and distances between 0 and 150 meters. Clofibric acid attains relatively low removal efficiency as compared to other blood lipid regulators. Regardless of travel times and distances, blood lipid regulators were removed above 50%; thus, MAR systems are effective for reducing blood lipid regulators even in short travel times and distances.

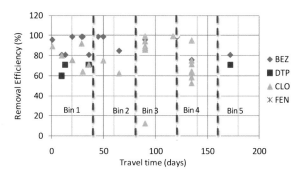

Figure 7.3 Plot of removal efficiency of blood lipid regulators with travel times

Table 7.8 Analysis of scatter plot of blood lipid regulators removal with travel times

Influent (ng/L)	Effluent (ng/L)	Time (days)	Removal (%)	Number of cases	Average (%)	Standard Deviation (%)	Predictive Removal (%)
0-60	0-5	0-40	60-99	17	81	13	57-68
		40-80	62-99	5	84	16	68-83
		80-120	13-99	9	85	28	83-92
		120-160	53-95	16	76	16	92-94
		160-200	71-81	2	76	7	>94

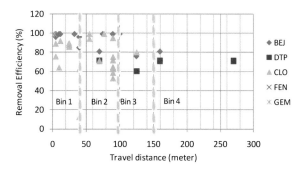

Figure 7.4 Plot of removal efficiency of blood lipid regulators with travel distances

Table 7.9 Analysis of scatter plot of blood lipid regulator removals with distances

Influent (ng/L)	Effluent (ng/L)	Distance (m)	Removal (%)	Number of cases	Average (%)	Standard Deviation (%)	Predictive Removal (%)
0-60	0-5	0-50	13-99	19	86	21	65-69
		50-100	62-99	28	80	15	69-83
		100-150	60-80	3	72	11	83-95
		>150	71-81	4	74	5	95-100

Analgesics

Diclofenac (DIC), indomethacin (IND), propyphenazone (PRO), naproxen (NAP), pentoxifyline (PEN), and ibuprofen (IBU) are analgesics that are very common PhACs that often detected from LBF sites (Lakes Tegel and Wannsee in Germany) (Heberer and Adam, 2004; Heberer et al., 2003b; Heberer et al., 2004; Heberer et al., 2003a; Massmann et al., 2006; Pekdeger, 2006; Verstraeten et al., 2002). Scatter plots of the removal efficiencies for analgesics with travel times and travel distances are presented below (Figure 7.5 and Figure 7.6) and the analyses are presented in Table 7.10 and Table 7.11. It can be noted that LBF removes analgesics greater than 60%, within residence times between 40 - 173 days and travel distance above 100 meters. Moreover, there were some correlations observed between analgesic removals and travel distances, in that the removal of analgesics increased with travel distances. Travel distance may play an important factor in controlling the removal of analgesics.

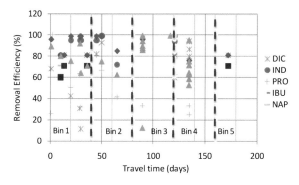

Figure 7.5 Plot of removal efficiency of analgesics with travel times

Table 7.10 Analysis of scatter plot of analgesics removal with travel times

Influent (ng/L)	Effluent (ng/L)	Time (days)	Removal (%)	Number of cases	Average (%)	Standard Deviation (%)	Predictive Removal (%)
0-485	0-301	0-40	8-99	28	71	28	43-64
		40-80	91-100	7	82	18	64-77
		80-120	93-99	20	82	14	77-96
		120-173	71-99	13	88	11	96-100

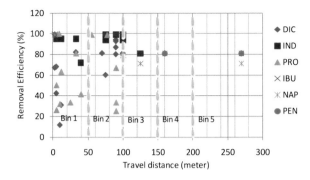

Figure 7.6 Plot of removal efficiency of analgesics with travel distances

Table 7.11 Analysis of scatter plot of analgesics removal with travel distances

Influent (ng/L)	Effluent (ng/L)	Distance (m)	Removal (%)	Number of cases	Average (%)	Standard Deviation (%)	Predictive Removal (%)
0-230	0-170	0-50	12-99	29	70	30	41-60
		50-100	25-81	19	81	22	60-72
		100-150	71-81	3	78	6	72-75
		150-200	81	5	79	4	75-83
		200-270	71-81	5	77	5	83-100

Anticonvulsants

Carbamazepine (CAR) and primidone (PRI) are commonly used for anticonvulsants (Heberer et al., 2003b; Heberer et al., 2004; Heberer et al., 2003a; Massmann et al., 2006; Mechlinski and Heberer, 2005; Pekdeger, 2006). Scatter plots of anticonvulsants with travel times and travel distances are presented Figure 7.7 and Figure 7.8 and the analyses of the scatter plot are shown in Table 7.12 and Table 7.13. It can be noted that most of the data points occur below 50% removal efficiency, within travel distances less than 50 meters and travel times less than 50 days. However, anticonvulsants appear to be reduced as travel times and travel distances increased. As shown in Figure 7.7 and Figure 7.8, in some cases, removals of anticonvulsants were removed up to 90%. In fact, previous studies have shown that carbamazepine and primidone were persistent compounds during wastewater or water treatment processes. The removal of anticonvulsants is due to mixing from native groundwater because the mixing with groundwater generally increases with travel times and distances. Therefore, more data are required to investigate if the removal of anticonvulsants is possible during MAR.

160

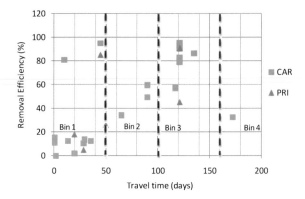

Figure 7.7 Plot of removal efficiency of anticonvulsants with travel times

Table 7.12 Analysis of scatter plot of anticonvulsants removal with travel times

Influent (ng/L)	Effluent (ng/L)	Time (days)	Removal (%)	Number of cases	Average (%)	Standard Deviation (%)	Predictive Removal (%)
0-583	5-520	0-40	0-81	11	16	22	0-30
		40-80	26-95	4	60	30	30-50
		80-120	49-60	3	55	5	50-54
		120-173	33-95	12	76	22	54-98

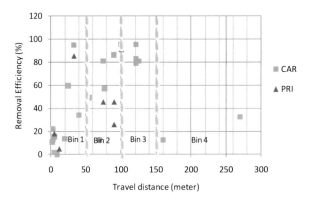

Figure 7.8 Plot of removal efficiency of anticonvulsants with travel distances

Table 7.13 Analysis of scatter plot of anticonvulsants removal with travel distances

Influent (ng/L)	Effluent (ng/L)	Distance (m)	Removal (%)	Number of cases	Average (%)	Standard Deviation	Predictive Removal (%)
0-583	5-520	0-50	2-95	16	27	28	0-8
		50-100	13-91	10	59	28	8-31
		100-150	79-95	4	85	7	31-77
		>150	13-33	2	23	14	77-92

Antibiotics

Sulfamethoxazole (SUL), acetyl sulfamethoxazole (ACS), clarithromycin (CLA), roxithromycin, clindamycin (CLI) and trimethoprim (TRI) were detected at LBF sites from Lake Tegel and Lake Wannsee, Berlin, Germany (Grunheid and Jekel, 2005; Grunheid et al., 2005; Heberer et al., 2008). Scatter plots of the removal efficiencies for antibiotics with travel times and travel distances are presented below in Figure 7.9 and Figure 7.10 and the analyses of the scatter plot are shown in Table 7.14 and Table 7.15. It can be noted that mostly the removal of antibiotics was not significant within residence times up to 40 days and distances less than 50 meters. However, antibiotics are removed as travel distances and residence time increased. All antibiotics were significantly attenuated after 3 months of travel times. Sulfamethoxazole, known to be a redox dependence compound, reduced as travel distances and travel times increased (Heberer et al., 2008). Generally, redox conditions become more reduced as travel distance and travel times increase. Therefore, redox conditions may also control the removal of sulfamethoxazole which was removed better under anoxic conditions.

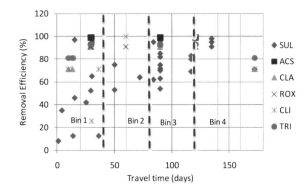

Figure 7.9 Plot of removal efficiency of antibiotics with travel times

Table 7.14 Analysis of scatter plot of antibiotics removal with travel time

Influent (ng/L)	Effluent (ng/L)	Time (days)	Removal (%)	Number of cases	Average (%)	Standard Deviation	Predictive Removal (%)
0-485	0-301	0-40	8-99	28	71	28	43-64
		40-80	91-100	7	82	18	64-77
		80-120	93-99	20	82	14	77-96
		120-173	71-99	13	88	11	96-100

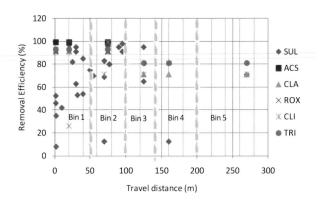

Figure 7.10 Plot of removal efficiency of antibiotics with travel distances

Table 7.15 Analysis of scatter plot of antibiotics removal with travel distances

Influent (ng/L)	Effluent (ng/L)	Distance (m)	Removal (%)	Number of cases	Average (%)	Standard Deviation	Predictive Removal (%)
0-485	0-301	0-50	8-99	35	78	25	54-62
		50-100	13-99	16	84	22	62-66
		100-150	65-95	7	76	10	66-69
		150-200	13-81	4	61	33	69-79
		200-270	71-81	4	74	5	79-94

Beta blockers

Atenolol (ATE), metoprolol (MET), bisoprolol (BIS) and sotalol (SOT) were detected from RBF sites located at river Rhine, Elbe and Ruhr (Germany) (Schmidt et al., 2007). Scatter plot of beta blockers with residence times and travel distances are presented below in Figure 7.10 and Figure 7.11. However, guidelines are not significant to predict the removal efficiency of beta blocker because of limited data available from the field studies mentioned above. Therefore, guidelines for beta blockers are not presented. However, Schimidt et al. (2007) showed that beta blockers such as ATE, MET and BIS were removed greater than 70% at RBF sites.

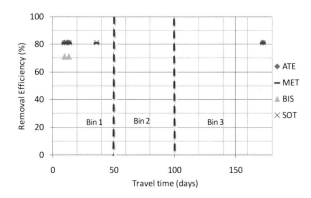

Figure 7.11 Plot of removal efficiency of beta blockers with travel times

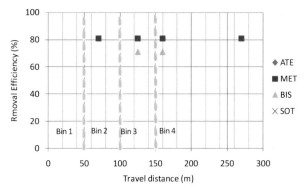

Figure 7.12 Plot of removal efficiency of beta blockers with travel distances

7.3.3. Development of water quality prediction tool

The proposed water quality predictive removal performances are incorporated into a simple Microsoft Excel spreadsheet to enable preliminary estimation of the removal of the different groups of OMPs; X-ray contrast agents, PhACs, EDCs, pesticides and volatile organic compounds. The tool is comprised of several worksheets that compute the guidelines basing on either a known residence time or well distance from surface water sources (e.g., lake, river and infiltration basin) (Figure 7.13, Figure 7.14 and Figure 7.15). The removal efficiencies estimated by the spreadsheet are however limited to the influent and effluent ranges for which these guidelines were developed (i.e., boundary conditions). The tool was also developed to give preliminary guidelines for the removal of dissolved organic carbon and six selected OMPs: phenazone (PhACs), propyphenazone (PhACs), acetylaminoantipyrine (AAA) (transformation product), formylaminoantipyrine (FAA) (transformation product), adsorbable organic bromide (AOBr) and carbamazepine. These removals were based on a first-order kinetics model estimated in the analysis of the NASRI data and can be applied under similar site conditions as that at the NASRI project sites (Figure 7.16).

The introduction/home page, typical computation worksheets and references of the water quality prediction tool are as shown in Figure 7.12, Figure 7.13 and Figure 7.14, respectively. On each computation sheet for the removal of groups of OMPs, the limits of the guidelines are clearly indicated and a hyperlink is provided for the full display of the guidelines and literature references used in their compilation.

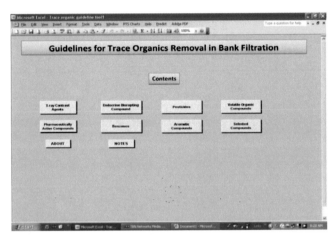

Figure 7.13 Introduction page of the water quality prediction tool

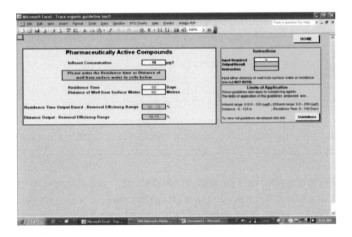

Figure 7.14 Typical computation worksheet for guidelines of a group of OMPs

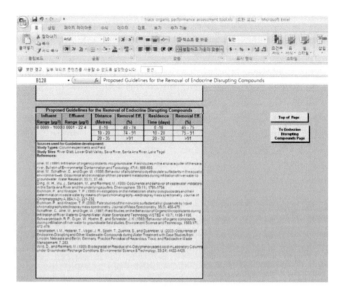

Figure 7.15 A list of references used for guideline developments

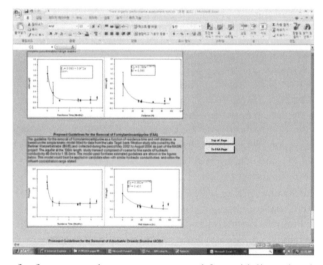

Figure 7.16 A list of references and rate constants used for guidelines development

Input Parameters

The input parameters for the preliminary estimation of the removal of groups of OMPs are:

- Influent concentration – The influent concentration of the surface water source is required mainly to confirm if the parameter fell within the stated influent range. This input is linked to a message cell that provides feedback on whether the OMP is within the range or not.
- Well distance from the surface water source (travel distance) – The expected/known distance of a well from the surface water source is a required input, especially if the residence time is not known. For a planned/non-existent MAR system, it is most likely that the residence/travel time at the site may not be known. The spreadsheet estimates are

computed based on either the well distances or the residence times. If both inputs are available, then two sets of results would be expected, which could then be compared.

- Travel time – The travel time of water from the surface water source to a given well location, is required as one of the inputs. This input requirement may be preferred to the previous variable as it is more representative of the actual flow path of contaminants.

As may be noted in Figure 7.13, the input requirements are indicated by yellow cells in the spreadsheet, while the outputs are indicated by blue cells. The green cells show instructions to be followed especially with regard to the influent concentration range.

Output Parameters

The output parameters of the estimation of removal of OMPs was basically a range of removal efficiencies, which were either based on the travel times or well distances. For the selected OMPs, outputs were given as both removal efficiencies and effluent concentrations. It should be noted that in both cases the removal efficiencies estimated are based on either travel times or travel distances. Hence, if both inputs are available/known, then the two sets of results can simply be compared, whereas if only one is known, at least one result would be expected. These outputs are simply a guide of the anticipated removals for a given MAR site.

Limitations

Some of the limitations in the use of this spreadsheet model/tool are listed below:

- It can only be used within the specified influent ranges, hence if a given site has influent concentrations outside this range, no preliminary estimates of removal can be determined.
- The predicted removal efficiencies were based on only travel times and well-surface water distances (travel distances), whereas there are several other important factors such as redox conditions, flow velocity, transmissivity, etc, which, if known and incorporated in the tool would improve the estimates.
- The treated water quality estimated for the selected OMPs, were based on kinetic models and a multi-regression model fitted to data from the Lake Tegel LBF site, which makes them quite specific. Hence, their use would be best applied in cases where site conditions such as aquifer material, transmissivity, redox conditions, etc, are generally similar.
- For a more fruitful use of this water quality prediction tool, general knowledge on the removal/persistent nature of a compound may be necessary, so as to avoid mis-interpreting the predicted guidelines. This is because not all compounds falling in a given group of OMPs may actually follow the predicted guideline/trend.

Some guidelines were developed with a relatively limited number of data points, hence narrowing the limits of the distances, residence times and influent ranges.

7.3.4. Quantitative structure activity relationship (QSAR) models based on field studies

A summary of developed QSAR models for PhACs, based on therapeutic usage, is shown in Table 7.16. A summary of selected descriptors is shown in Table 7.17. Travel time (TIME) appears in most of QSAR models, and is an important parameter for RBF systems with respect to OMPs removal (Schmidt et al., 2007). Validation of the models was not carried out because this evaluation was to investigate the most important parameters explaining the removal of selected PhACs during soil passage. Table 7.18 shows an example of estimated descriptors for some PhACs.

Table 7.16 Summary of QSAR models for PhACs removal based on therapeutic usage

Group	Model Equation	R^2
Analgesics	% Removal = 572.421 X4Av -3.489 nCp - 1.399 nCbH + 59.802	0.76
Antibiotics	% Removal = 0.194 TIME + 11.805 KOWEX+ 29.978B2 + 42.238	0.34
Beta Blockers	% Removal = 0.039 TIME - 4.646 nCp + 91.124	0.91
Anticonvulsants	% Removal = 0.426 TIME +18.09	0.40
X-ray contrast agents	% Removal = 0.094 TIME - 12.444 nCp + 8.376 nROH+ 76.637	0.64
Steroid hormones	% Removal = 0.003 DIST + 99.09	0.99
Anti depressants	% Removal = 3431.769 X4Av + 9.064	0.85
Blood lipid regulators	% Removal = 0.062 TIME + 35.096 B1 + 57.078	0.75

Table 7.17 Summary of selected descriptors for field study

Descriptors		Type
TIME	Residence times	Operation conditions
DIST	Travel distances	Operation conditions
X4Av	Average valence connectivity index	Connectivity indices
nCp	Number of terminal primary carbon	Functional groups
nCbH	Number of unsubstituted benzene	Functional groups
KOWEX	log K_{ow} (n-octanol/water partition coefficient)	Physicochemical properties
nROH	Number of hydroxyl groups	Functional groups
B1	Biodegradation potential from linear model*	Biodegradation potential
B2	Biodegradation potential from non-linear model*	Biodegradation potential

* BIOWIN, US EPA 2009 Estimation programs interface suite[TM] for MS windows

Table 7.18 Example of descriptor estimations

		X4Av	nCp	nCbH	nROH
Analgesics	Ibuprofen	1.556	3	4	1
Blood lipid regulators	Bezafibrate	2.212	2	8	1
Anticonvulsants	Carbamazepine	2.211	80	8	0

7.3.5. Quantitative structure activity relationship model developed in laboratory-scale study

Model Development

Reliable data of PhACs are needed to develop a model that can be explained in a mechanistic manner. Having results under different spatial and hydrogeochemical conditions (i.e, field studies) will easily lead to a model with limited applicability. In this study, experimental data from column studies using four different classes of PhACs including lipid regulators, psychostimulants, analgesics and anticonvulsants (13 selected PhACs) were used for developing a QSAR model. Adding more cases from the different therapeutic usages of PhACs (e.g., antibiotics) would certainly increase the applicability of the model. Genetic algorithm was used to select the best descriptors followed by an ordinary least squares (OLS) method to develop the QSAR model. Genetic algorithms (GA) are an evolutionary method which often used in several fields such as chemistry and QSAR (Goldberg, 1989). GA selects descriptors by considering populations of models generated through a reproduction process and optimized according to a given objectives (Todeschini et al., 2003). The model was selected based on the correlation coefficient (R^2) and the external predictivity. The following QSAR model based on 4 variables was selected among 247 molecular descriptors.

% removal of PhACs = 174.8($\pm$11.6) nImidazoles + 158.4($\pm$19.8) AR $-$ 98.1($\pm$5.8) nCONN $-$ 1830.3($\pm$193.2) ME + 1851.1($\pm$188.3)

$R^2 = 0.84$, $Q^2 = 0.81$ and $Q^2_{ext} = 0.64$

Number of cases in the training set = 65, number of cases in the testing set = 26 cases (external validation)

As shown in Table 7.19, there are four variables selected in the model (NImidazloles, AR, nCONN and ME) to estimate the removal of PhACs tested in the column studies. Selected descriptors with positive coefficients indicate that those descriptors contribute positively to the removal of PhACs, whereas descriptors with negative coefficients lead to an inverse effect on PhACs removal. During soil column experiments, ionic PhACs were not effectively removed under abiotic conditions using sodium azide (abiotic conditions where only sorption is influential) but were significantly removed under biotic conditions. Moreover, physicochemical properties associated with sorption and electrostatic forces (e.g., dipole moment, K_{ow}, etc.) had little or no impact on the model. Therefore, it is believed that the selected descriptors may correlate to biodegradation. The significance of the selected descriptors can be determined using standardized regression coefficient values; ME (Mean atomic Sanderson Electronegativity) (-0.8) and AR (aromatic ratio) (0.8) in the model are relatively low compared to nCONN (-1.6) and nImidazoles (2.5). All variables have different units of measurements, and these variables were standardized by subtracting the mean and dividing by the standard deviation. ME was selected in the model because it indicates the negative influence of electronegativity of PhACs. On the other hand, an increase in the number of Imidazole groups (i.e., functional groups) leads to an increase in biodegradation. According to Organization for Economic Co-operation and Development (OECD) Screening Information DataSet (SIDS) report, imidazole is a readily biodegradable compound that degrades between 90 and 100% (OECD, 2003). nCONN was probably selected because carbamazepine, the most persistent compound during the soil passage, contains urea derivatives. Table 7.20 shows an example of estimated descriptors for some PhACs.

Table 7.19 Summary of selected descriptors

	Descriptors	Type	
NImidazloles	Number of Imidazole groups	Functional groups	
AR	Aromatic ratio (number of aromatic bond over the total Number of non-H bonds)	Constitutional descriptors	
nCONN	number of urea (-thio) derivatives	Functional group	
ME	Mean atomic Sanderson electronegativity (scaled on carbon atom)	Constitutional descriptors	

Table 7.20 Example of descriptor estimations

		NImidazoles	AR	nCONN	ME
Analgesics	Ibuprofen	0	0.4	0	0.9
Blood lipid regulators	Gemfibrozil	0	0.3	0	0.9
Anticonvulsants	Carbamazepine	0	0.6	1	1

Model validation

R^2 is often used as a measure of goodness-of-fit of a QSAR model. However, validation has to be carried out to determine the robustness and predictivity of the model. LOO cross validation, the most commonly applied for an internal validation, was used to predict the reliability of the model (Gramatica, 2007). Thus, if the cross validation coefficient Q^2 is greater than 0.5, then the model can be attributed a high predictive power (Ghasemi et al., 2009). The developed QSAR model presented a Q^2 of 0.81. Therefore, the model was acceptable by analyzing LOO cross validation.

External data collected from various field studies were used for external validation of the QSAR model. According to Gramatica (2007), only externally validated models are applicable to both external prediction and regulatory purposes. A Q^2_{ext} value of 0.64 was obtained, suggesting the prediction power of the model by external validation was lower than that of internal validation.

7.4. Conclusions

The framework for assessment of OMP removals for MAR systems (guidelines and QSAR models) developed from this study could be a useful tool to provide more understanding of the behavior of OMPs during soil passage. The proposed guidelines deal with different classes of OMPs and suggest removal efficiencies of the pollutants as function of travel times and travel distances. In this study, travel times and travel distances appear to be good parameters in estimating PhACs removal for MAR systems. However, travel times appear to be better compared to travel distances to estimate the removal of PhACs. Different types of molecular descriptors (constitutional descriptors, connectivity indices and functional groups) were used for the development of QSAR models to understand the fate of PhACs during soil passage. Sorption properties associated with chemical, physical and electrostatic forces (e.g., log D, dipole moment, log K_{ow}, etc.) had little or no impact on the model. Therefore, it is likely that the selected descriptors are correlated to biodegradation. More data on removal of different types of PhACs would enhance the applicability of the model. Moreover, different QSAR models for ionic and non-ionic PhACs will further improve the prediction power of the models. The framework for assessment of OMP removals would be useful to water utilities for adapting MAR as a multi-objective (-contaminant) barrier and understanding different classes of compounds, and it would also help to determine post treatment requirements for MAR.

Based on the data analysis, guidelines and QSAR models developed during this study the following conclusions can be made:

- Preliminary guidelines developed can be used as a screening tool to assess removal of OMPs for MAR systems under given conditions.

- Based on PhACs guidelines, antibiotics, analgesics, beta blockers and steroid hormones are generally removed efficiently during soil passage (from 50 to 90%).

- As persistent compounds, the attenuation of anticonvulsants observed during MAR (40 to 50%) was may be due to mixing from native groundwater.

- The developed QSAR model links important physicochemical properties to the removal of OMPs, and the models are useful to predict the fate of a new compound during soil passage.

- Travel time was found to be an important variable that contributes to the removal of PhACs. Thus, removal efficiency of PhACs during MAR can be increased by enhancing the travel time.

- QSAR model developed from laboratory scale experiment included ME (Mean atomic Sanderson Electronegativity), AR (aromatic ratio), nCONN (number of urea (-thio) derivatives) and nImidazoles (number of Imidazole) for descriptors that predict the performance of simulated MAR system.

- It was observed that the development of a QSAR model is highly dependent on quality of data used. Each MAR site has different characteristics including hydrogeochemical conditions, travel distances, travel times etc. Moreover, the proper selection of the molecular descriptors that define or correlate with different mechanisms taking place during MAR is very important to get a representative QSAR model.

7.5. References

Cambridge, 2002. Soft Corporation, CS Chem3D Ultra 7.0, USA, http://www.cambridgesoft.com/.

Díaz-Cruz M.S. and Barceló D., 2008. Trace organic chemicals contamination in ground water recharge. Chemosphere 72, 333-342.

Goldberg D.E. 1989. Genetic algorithms in search, optimization and machine learning, Addison-Wesley, Massachusetts, MA

Ghasemi J.B., Abdolmaleki A. and Mandoumi N., 2009. A quantitative structure property relationship for prediction of solubilization of hazardous compounds using GA-based MLR in CTAB micellar media. J. Hazard. Mater. 161, 74-80.

Gramatica P., 2007 Principles of QSAR models validation: internal and external. QSAR Comb. Sci. 26, 694-701.

Grunheid S. and Jekel M., 2005. Fate of trace organic pollutants during bank filtration and groundwater recharge, 5th International Symposium on Management of Aquifer Recharge, 10-16 June 2005, Berlin, Germany.

Grunheid S., Amy G. and Jekel M., 2005. Removal of bulk dissolved organic carbon (DOC) and trace organic compounds by bank filtration and artificial recharge. Water Res. 39, 3219-3228.

Heberer T., Adam M., 2004. Transport and Attenuation of Pharmaceutical Residues During Artificial Groundwater Replenishment. Environ. Chem. 1, 22-25.

Heberer T., Mechlinski A., Fanck B., 2003b. NASRI - Occurrence and Fate of Pharmaceuticals during Bank Filtration, Conference Wasser Berlin 2003, Berlin Centre for Water Competence, Berlin.

Heberer T., Massmann G., Fanck B., Taute T., Dünnbier U., 2008. Behaviour and redox sensitivity of antimicrobial residues during bank filtration. Chemosphere 73, 451-460.

Heberer T., Mechlinski A., Fanck B., Knappe A., Massmann G., Pekdeger A., Fritz B., 2004. Field Studies on the Fate and Transport of Pharmaceutical Residues in Bank Filtration. Ground Water Monit. R., 24, 70-77.

Heberer T., Fanck B., Mechlinski A., Zühlke S., Adam M., Voigt M., Wicke D., Dünnbier U., 2003a. Occurrence and Fate of Drug Residues and Related Polar Contaminants during Bank Filtration, Berlin Centre for Water Competence, Berlin.

Hiscock K.M., Grischek T., 2002. Attenuation of groundwater pollution by bank filtration. J. Hydrol. 266, 139-144.

Massmann G., Greskowiak J., Dünnbier U., Zuehlke S., Knappe A., Pekdeger A., 2006. The impact of variable temperatures on the redox conditions and the behaviour of pharmaceutical residues during artificial recharge. J. Hydrol. 328, 141-156.

Mechlinski A., Heberer T., 2005. Fate and transport of pharmaceutical residues during bank filtration, 5th international symposium on management of aquifer recharge, 10-16 June 2005, UNESCO, Berlin, Germany.

OECD, 2003. SIDS Initial Assessment Report for SIAM 17. UNEP PUBLICATIONS. http://www.inchem.org/documents/sids/sids/288324.pdf. Accessed 07 January 2010.

Pekdeger A., 2006. Hydrogeological-hydrogeochemical processes during bank filtration and groundwater recharge using a mulit-tracer approach, NASRI Project, Berlin.

Ray C., 2008. Worldwide potential of riverbank filtration. Clean Techn. Environ. Policy 10, 223-225.

Ray C., Soong T.W., Lian Y.Q., Roadcap G.S., 2002. Efffect of flood-induced chemical load on filtrate quality at bank filtration sites. J. Hydrol. 266, 235-258.

Scheytt T., Mersmann P., Leidig M., Pekdeger A., Heberer T., 2004. Transport of Pharmaceutically Active Compounds in Saturated Laboratory Columns. Ground Water 42, 767-773.

Schmidt C.K., Lange F.T., Brauch H.J., 2007 Characteristics and evaluation of natural attenuation processes for organic micropollutant removal during riverbank filtration, Regional IWA conference on groundwater management in the Danube River Basin and other large River Basins, 7-9 June 2007, Belgrade, Serbia.

Schmidt C.K., Lange F.T., Brauch H.J., W. K., 2003. Experiences with riverbank filtration and infiltration in Germany, International symposium on artificial recharge of groundwater, K-WATER, Daejon, Korea.

Talete., 2009. MobyDigs – software for multilinear regression analysis and variable subset selection by genetic algorithm, in: Version 1.1 http://www.talete.mi.it/.

Tao S., Xi X., Xu F., Dawson R., 2002. A QSAR model for predicting toxicity (LC50) to rainbow trout. Water Res. 36, 2926-2930.

Todeschini R., Consonni V., Mauri A., Pavan M., 2003. MOBYDIGS: software for regression and classification model by genetic algorithms. In: Leardi R. (Ed.). Nature-inspired methods in chemometrics: genetic algorithms and artificial neural networks. Elsevier, B.V., Amsterdam, The Netherlands.

US EPA., 2009. Estimation Programs Interface Suite™ for Microsoft® Windows, v 4.00, United States Environmental Protection Agency, Washington, DC, USA.

Verstraeten I.M., Heberer T., Scheytt T., 2002 Occurrence, characteristics, and transport and fate of pesticides, pharmaceutical active compounds, and industrial and personal care products at bank-filtration sites, Riverbank Filtration: Improving Source-Water Quality, Kluwer Academic Publishers, Dordrecht.

Walker J.D., Jaworska J., Comber M.H., Schultz T.W., Dearden J.C., 2003. Guidelines for developing and using quantitative structure-activity relationships. Environ. Toxicol. Chem. 22, 1653-1665.

Yangali-Quintanilla V., Sadmani A., McConville M., Kennedy M., Amy G., 2010. A QSAR model for predicting rejection of emerging contaminants (pharmaceuticals, endocrine disruptors) by nanofiltration membranes. Water Res. 44, 373-384.

Chapter 8

SUMMARY AND CONCLUSIONS

8.1. Bank filtration: potential and challenge

Natural treatment systems such as bank filtration (BF) (i.e., managed aquifer recharge)) are robust barriers for many organic micropollutants (OMPs) and may represent a low-cost alternative compared to advanced drinking water treatment systems. BF has been successfully applied for water treatment in Europe and United States, and many water utilities companies have a great interest in BF as a new source of water supply. However, existing BF facilities have all been based on local experiences. For water supply companies, currently there are no tools or guidelines for the design of BF systems and prediction of the fate of pharmaceutical active compounds (PhACs) or endocrine disrupting compounds (EDCs) during soil passage.

One of the objectives of this thesis was to understand and to develop tools to utilize the multiple objective water treatment potential of BF for wastewater effluent-impacted surface water. This study mainly focused on the removal of bulk organic matter, EDCs and PhACs. This study focused on the following specific objectives: (i) an evaluation of the changes in the character of bulk organic matter upon soil column passage to simulate the impact of wastewater effluent during BF, (ii) an understanding of the fate of EDCs and selected PhACs during BF, and (iii) an investigation of selected OMPs with hydrogeochemical conditions and spatial parameters using principal component analysis in order to statistically delineate removal trends at BF and AR sites. A framework or guidelines for the assessment or prediction of OMP removals from a BF system will be an important tool for quick screening of candidate BF project sites and to compare performance costs with other conventional treatment systems. This study involved of soil column and batch reactors experiments in the laboratory and a field study carried out from Berlin, Germany.

8.2. Occurrence and fate of bulk organic matter and PhACs in managed aquifer recharge

Detailed characteristics of bulk organic matter and the occurrence and fate of PhACs during through managed aquifer recharge (MAR) treatment processes such as BF and AR were reviewed. Understanding the fate of bulk organic matter through BF and AR is essential to determine the pre- and/or post-treatment requirements. Organic matter characteristic results obtained using a suite of analytical tools suggests that there was a preferential removal of non-humic substances. Different classes of PhACs behave differently during BF and AR. Antibiotics, non-steroidal anti-inflammatory drugs (NSAIDs), beta blockers and steroid hormones generally exhibited good removal efficiencies, especially for compounds having hydrophobic-neutral characteristics. However, anticonvulsants showed a persistent behavior during soil passage. There were also some redox dependent PhACs. For example, X-Ray contrast agents, determined as adsorbable organic iodine (AOI), and sulfamethoxazole (antibiotics) was degraded more favorably under anoxic conditions compared to oxic conditions. Phenazone-type pharmaceuticals (NSAIDs) exhibited better removal efficiencies under oxic conditions. The redox transition from oxic to anoxic conditions during soil passage can enhance the removal of PhACs that are sensitive to redox conditions. BF and AR can potentially be included in a multi-barrier treatment system for the removal of PhACs.

8.3. Fate of effluent organic matter during bank filtration

Understanding the fate of effluent organic matter (EfOM) and natural organic matter (NOM) through BF is essential to assess the impact of wastewater effluent on the post treatment requirements of bank filtrates. EfOM includes humic substances which are derived from the drinking water source and serve as a precursor to disinfection by-product (DBPs) while SMPs (proteins) in EfOM represent a precursor to nitrogenous DBPs (N-DBPs). Column studies were conducted to characterize bulk organic matter which consists of EfOM and NOM during BF using a suite of innovative analytical tools and determine the removal of selected PhACs. Results showed the preferential removal of non-humic substances (i.e., biopolymers) from wastewater effluent-impacted surface water. The bulk organic matter characteristics of wastewater effluent-impacted surface water and surface water were similar after 5 m soil passage. Humic-like organic matter in surface water and wastewater effluent-impacted surface water persisted through soil passage. More than 50% of dissolved organic carbon (DOC) removal with significant reduction of dissolved oxygen (DO) was observed in the top 50 cm of the soil columns. This was due to biodegradation by soil biomass which was determined by adenosine triphosphate (ATP) concentrations and heterotrophic plate counts. Good correlation of DOC removal with DO and biomass development was observed in the soil columns. DOC removal was reduced under anoxic conditions compared to oxic conditions. Most of the selected PhACs exhibited removal efficiencies of greater than 90% in both wastewater effluent-dominated surface water and surface water. However, removal efficiencies of bezafibrate, diclofenac, and gemfibrozil were relatively low in wastewater effluent-impacted surface water which appears to have more biodegradable organic carbon (BDOC) from EfOM. This result indicates that BDOC characteristics or microbial diversity affect the biotransformation of some PhACs. Further study is needed to define the microorganisms responsible for biotransformation of the PhACs. Carbamazepine and clofibric acid showed a persistent behavior and were not influenced by EfOM. The removal efficiencies of selected PhACs in this study did not vary under different redox conditions.

8.4. Fate of endocrine disrupting compounds during bank filtration

With rapid development in technology and instrumentation, researchers are able to measure emerging trace contaminants more accurately and EDCs have been recognized as a new category of environmental contaminants that interrupt the function of the endocrine system. The feminization of male aquatic species in receiving waters mainly originated from effluents from wastewater treatment plants, and surface runoff from agricultural activities and municipal biosolids. It is important to investigate the fate of EDCs during BF. Laboratory-scale batch and soil columns experiments were conducted to determine the primary mechanisms of EDCs (estrogen compounds) and identify factors need to be important to consider for the removal of estrogen compounds. Biotic and abiotic experiments were also employed using batch experiment to investigate the role of microbial activity in the removal of estrogen compounds. Moreover, different redox conditions in batch experiment were also conducted under different redox conditions to investigate the impact of different redox conditions on the estrogen removals. Based on the results of this study, adsorption and biodegradation are important removal mechanisms, but adsorption was revealed as the primary removal mechanism. 17-estradiol and 17-ethinylestradiol were removed 99% and 96%, respectively, in batch experiments. Factors considered in this study (i.e., microbial activity associated with sand and redox conditions) did not reveal effects on the removal of 17-estradiol. However, 17-ethinylestradiol removals varied from 64% to 87% for the columns prepared for different degrees of biodegradation.

8.5. Role of biodegradation in the removal of PhACs during bank filtration

Natural treatment systems such BF have been recognized as an effective barrier in the multi-barrier approach for the attenuation of organic micropollutants for safe drinking water supply. In this study, the role of biodegradation in removing selected PhACs during soil passage was investigated. Batch studies were first conducted to investigate the removal of 13 selected PhACs from different water sources with respect to different sources of biodegradable organic matter. Column experiments were then performed to differentiate between biodegradation and sorption in the removal of selected PhACs. Selected neutral PhACs (phenacetine, paracetamol and caffeine) and acidic PhACs (ibuprofen, fenoprofen, bezafibrate and naproxen) exhibited removal efficiencies of greater than 87% from different organic water matrices during batch studies (contact time: 60 days). In column studies, removal efficiencies of acidic PhACs (i.e., analgesics) decreased under biodegradable carbon-limited conditions. Removal efficiencies of selected acidic PhACs (ibuprofen, fenoprofen, bezafibrate, ketoprofen and naproxen) were less than 35% under abiotic conditions. This was attributed to sorption under abiotic conditions established by a biocide (20 mM of sodium azide), which suppressed microbial activity/biodegradation. However, under biotic conditions, removal efficiencies of these acidic PhACs compounds were greater than 78%, mainly attributed to biodegradation. Moreover, average removal efficiencies of hydrophilic (polar) neutral PhACs with low octanol/water partition coefficients (log K_{ow} < 2) (paracetamol, pentoxifylline, phenacetine and caffeine) were low (< 12 %) under abiotic conditions. However, under biotic conditions, removal efficiencies of selected neutral PhACs were greater than 91%. In contrast, carbamazepine showed a persistent behavior in both batch and column studies. Overall, this study found that biodegradation was an important mechanism for the removal of PhACs during soil passage

8.6. Organic micropollutants removal from wastewater effluent-impacted drinking water sources during bank filtration and artificial recharge

Natural treatment systems such as BF and AR (via an infiltration basin) are a robust barrier for many OMPs and may represent a low-cost alternative compared to advanced drinking water treatment systems. This study analyzes a comprehensive database of OMPs at BF and AR sites located near Lake Tegel in Berlin (Germany). The focus of the study was on the derivation of correlations between the removal efficiencies of OMPs and key factors influencing the performance of BF and AR. At the BF site, shallow monitoring wells located close to the Lake Tegel source exhibited oxic conditions followed by prolonged anoxic conditions in deep monitoring wells and a more distant production well. At the AR site, oxic conditions prevailed from the recharge pond along monitoring wells to the production well. Long residence times of up to 4.5 months at the BF site reduced the temperature variation during soil passage between summer and winter. The temperature variations were greater at the AR site as a consequence of shorter residence times. Deep monitoring wells and the production well located at the BF site were under the influence of ambient groundwater and old bank filtrate (up to several years of age). Thus, it is important to account for mixing with native groundwater and other sources (e.g., old bank filtrate) when estimating the performance of BF with respect to removal of OMPs. Principal component analysis (PCA) was used to investigate correlations between OMP removals and hydrogeochemical conditions with spatial and temporal parameters (e.g., well distance, residence time and depth) from both sites. Principal component-1 (PC1) embodied redox conditions (oxidation reduction potential and dissolved oxygen), and principal component-2 (PC2) embodied degradation potential (e.g., total organic carbon and dissolved organic carbon) with the calcium carbonate dissolution potential (Ca^{2+} and HCO_3^-) for the BF site. These two PCs explained a total variance of 55% at the BF site. At the AR site, PCA revealed redox conditions (PC1) and degradation potential with temperature (PC2) as principal components, which explained a total variance of 56%.

8.7. Framework for assessment of organic micropollutants during managed aquifer recharge

MAR (e.g., BF and AR) is a reliable and proven process, in which water quality can be improved by different physical, biological, and chemical reactions during soil passage. As mentioned above, MAR can potentially be included in a multi-barrier treatment system for OMP removal in drinking water treatment and wastewater reuse schemes. However, there is a need to develop assessment tools to help implement MAR as an effective barrier in attenuating different OMPs including PhACs and EDCs. In this study, guidelines were developed for different classes of organic micropollutants, in which removal efficiencies of these compounds are determined as a function of travel times and distances. Guidelines are incorporated into Microsoft Excel spreadsheets and a simple water quality prediction tool was developed to estimate the removal of different classes of OMPs in MAR systems. Multiple linear regression analysis of data obtained from literature studies showed that travel time is one of the main parameters in estimating the performance of a MAR system for PhACs removal. Moreover, a quantitative structure activity relationship (QSAR) based model was proposed to predict the removals of OMPs. The QSAR approach is especially useful for compounds with little information about their fate during soil passage. Such an assessment framework for OMP removal is useful for adapting MAR as a multi-objective (-contaminant) barrier and understanding the fate of different classes of compounds during soil passage and the determination of post treatment requirements for MAR.

8.8. Practical implications of the finding and further research

Based on the findings of this study, BF is an effective barrier in the multi-barrier approach for removing organic micropollutants for safe drinking water supply. The removal efficiencies of BF for these contaminants can be maximised by proper design of the wells taking into consideration source water quality characteristics and local hydrogeological conditions. For practical implication of this study, most organic micropollutants can be removed during bank filtration, although to varying extents. More than 50% of bulk organic matter reduced within the first few meters. However, from the analysis of the guidelines developed in this study, the general observation noted for the groups of organic micropollutants selected in this study was that a minimum distance of 55 meters would achieve at least a 50% removal. With the exception of x-ray contrast agents and PhACs which showed a much higher range of residence times, the other groups generally showed residence times of least 20 days could achieve a minimum removal of 50%. It is also important to have enough residence time (e.g., 60 days) during BF in order to achieve biologically stable (biostable) bank filtrates (i.e., low assimilable organic carbon and microorganisms free). However, this could be a problem for some places where natural groundwater is contaminated because far from the river more landside groundwater will be part of bank filtrates. Generally, Oxic conditions followed by anoxic conditions during soil passage, and different redox conditions are effective for removing redox sensitive organic micropollutants during BF. One important conclusion of this study is that managed aquifer recharge such as BF alone is not capable of removing all organic micropollutants; therefore, it is important to choose the right post treatment process which maximize the removal of organic micropollutants. BF (i.e., managed aquifer recharge) followed by nanofiltration is an effective combination that will remove organic micropollutants first by biodegradation or by the membrane through mechanisms of size exclusion and charge repulsion. Although biodegradation, adsorption and mixing with natural groundwater achieve reduction of OMPs during managed aquifer recharge, the best solution for attenuating PhACs will be to avoid or minimize the use of organic micropollutants in a household and to adapt an advanced wastewater treatment processes such as membrane bioreactor for controlling point sources.

The developed guidelines for the groups of organic micropollutants can be further improved to increase their reliability, by including more literature sources than what was used to create the guidelines in this study. Detail studies on possible direct uptake of PhACs by microorganisms as a carbon source is necessary if PhACs are not always transformed by co-metabolism. Further research is necessary to investigate the fate of organic micropollutants during soil passage using different types of soil. More research should be carried out on the combination of managed aquifer recharge with other advanced water treatment processes (e.g., advanced oxidation and ion exchange systems). This would allow drinking water utilities to help identify the best combination of water treatment processes for removing organic micropollutants.

SAMENVATTING

Oeverfiltratie: potentieel en uitdaging

Natuurlijke zuiveringsprocessen, zoals oeverfiltratie (BF) (dwz, het kunstmatig aanvullen van aquifers)) vormen robuuste barrieres voor veel organische microverontreinigingen (OMPs) en kan een low-cost alternatief ten opzichte van geavanceerde technieken voor de behandeling van drinkwater. BF is met succes toegepast voor waterzuivering in Europa en de Verenigde Staten, en veel waterbedrijven hebben een grote interesse in BF als een nieuwe bron voor dinkwater. Echter, de bestaande BF faciliteiten zijn allemaal gebaseerd op lokale ervaringen. Voor de waterbedrijven zijn er momenteel geen middelen of richtlijnen voor het ontwerp van de BF-systemen en/of voor de voorspelling van het lot van farmaceutische actieve verbindingen (PhACs) of hormoonverstorende stoffen (EDC's) tijdens bodempassage.

Een van de doelstellingen van dit proefschrift was om het meerledige zuiveringspotentieel van BF te begrijpen en om instrumenten te ontwikkelen om dit potentieel meer te gebruiken voor de zuivering van oppervlaktewater, welke onder invloed staat van afvalwater. Deze studie is hoofdzakelijk gericht op de verwijdering van organische stof, EDC en PhACs. Dit onderzoek was gericht op de volgende specifieke doelstellingen: (i) een evaluatie van de veranderingen in het karakter van bulk organische stof tijdens bodempassage in een kolom om de impact van afvalwaterlozingen op BF te simuleren. (ii) een goed begrip van het lot van EDC en geselecteerde PhACs tijdens BF, en (iii) een onderzoek van geselecteerde OMPs met hydrogeochemische omstandigheden en ruimtelijke parameters met behulp van principale componenten analyse om statistisch verwijdering van OMPs tijdens BF en kunstmatige aanvulling (AR) af te bakenen.. Een kader of richtlijnen voor de beoordeling of de voorspelling van OMP verwijdering tijdens een BF-systeem, zal een belangrijk instrument vormen voor een snelle screening van mogelijke-BF oevers, en om de bij de prestatie horende kosten met andere conventionele zuiverinssystemen te vergelijken. Deze studie bestand uit kolomonderzoek en potjesproeven in het laboratorium en een veldonderzoek uitgevoerd vanuit Berlijn, Duitsland.

Voorkomen en lot van bulk organisch materiaal en PhACs tijdens het kunstmatig aanvullen van aquifers

Gedetailleerde eigenschappen van bulk organische stof en het voorkomen en het lot van PhACs tijdens kunstmatige aanvulling van aquifers (MAR) zuiveringsprocesses, zoals BF en AR, zijn besproken. Inzicht in het lot van bulk organische stof door middel van BF en AR is van essentieel belang om nodige voor en nabehandeling te kunnen vaststellen. Organische stof karakteristieke resultaten verkregen met behulp van een pakket aan analytische tools suggereerde dat er sprake was van een voorkeur voor de verwijdering van niet-humusachtige stoffen. Verschillende klassen van PhACs gedragen zich anders tijdens BF en AR. Antibiotica, niet-steroïdale anti-inflammatoire geneesmiddelen (NSAID's), bètablokkers en steroïd hormonen toonden in het algemeen een goede verwijdering, met name voor verbindingen met hydrofoob-neutrale kenmerken. Echter, anti-epileptica toonden hardnekkig gedrag tijdens bodempassage. Sommige PhAcs bleken redox afhankelijk. Bijvoorbeeld, rontgencontrastmiddelen, bepaald als absorbeerbare organische jodium (AOI), en sulfamethoxazol (antibiotica) werd beter afgebroken in zuurstofloze omstandigheden vergeleken met zuurstofrijke condities. Phenazone-achtige geneesmiddelen (NSAID's) lieten een betere verwijdering zien tijdens oxische omstandigheden. De overgang van oxische naar anoxische condities tijdens bodempassage is bevorderlijk voor de verwijdering van PhACs die gevoelig zijn voor redoxcondities. BF en AR kunnen mogelijk worden opgenomen in een multi-barrière systeem voor de verwijdering van PhACs.

Het lot van effluent organische stof tijdens oeverfiltratie

Inzicht in het lot van het effluent organische stof (EfOM) en natuurlijk organisch materiaal (NOM) tijdens BF is van essentieel belang om de benodigde nazuivering van oeverfiltraat te beoordelen. EfOM bevat humusstoffen die zijn te herleiden tot de drinkwaterbron en dienen als een voorspeller van desinfectie bijproducten (DBPs), terwijl SMP's (eiwitten) in EfOM een voorspeller zijn voor stikstofhoudende DBPs (N-DBPs).

Kolomondezoek werd uitgevoerd om bulk organische stof tijdens BF te karakteriseren, welke uit EfOM en NOM. Dit door het gebruik van een combinatie van innovatieve analytische tools en de verwijdering van geselecteerde PhACs te bepalen. De resultaten toonden een voorkeur aan voor de verwijdering van niet-humusachtige stoffen (dat wil zeggen, biopolymeren) uit oppervlakte water onder invloed van afvalwater effluent én van oppervlaktewater wasgelijk na 5 m bodempassage. Humus-achtige organische stof in het oppervlaktewater en oppervlaktewater onder invloed van afvalwater effluent bleken persistent tijdens bodem passage. Meer dan 50% van de opgeloste organische koolstof (DOC) verwijdering, met een significante vermindering van de opgeloste zuurstof (DO), werd waargenomen in de bovenste 50 cm van de kolommen. Dit was te wijten aan afbraak door de in de bodem aanwezige biomassa, welke werd bepaald door adenosine trifosfaat (ATP) concentraties en heterotrofe plaattellingen. Goede correlatie van DOC-verwijdering met DO en biomassa ontwikkeling werd waargenomen in de kolommen. DOC-verwijdering was minder onder zuurstofloze omstandigheden in vergelijking met zuurstof rijke omstandigheden.

De meeste van de geselecteerde PhACs lieten een verwijderingsrendement zien van meer dan 90%, in zowel oppervlaktewater als het oppervlaktewater onder invloed van afvalwatereffluent. Echter, het rendement van de verwijdering van bezafibraat, diclofenac en gemfibrozil waren relatief laag in het oppervlaktewater onder invloed van afvalwater. Terwijl de laatste waarschijnlijk meer biologisch afbreekbare organische koolstof (BDOC) heeft afkomstig van EfOM. Dit resultaat geeft aan dat ofwel de BDOC kenmerken of anders de microbiële diversiteit van invloed zijn op de biotransformatie van sommige PhACs. Nader onderzoek is nodig om de micro-organismen te definiëren welke verantwoordelijk zijn voor biotransformatie van het PhACs. Carbamazepine en clofibrinezuur toonden persistent gedrag en de verwijdering van deze PhAC's werd niet beïnvloed door EfOM. In deze studie is geen verschil in verwideringsrendement gevonden onder verschillende redox condities..

Het lot van de hormoonverstorende stoffen tijdens oeverfiltratie

Met de snelle ontwikkelingen in de technologie en meetinstrumenten zijn onderzoekers in staat om sporen van verontreinigingen zeer nauwkeuriger te meten.   Er worden ook hormonen en hormoonverstorende stoffen (EDC's) gemeten. Er zijn voorbeelden bekend waarbij mannelijke vissen vrouwelijke kenmerken ontwikkelen, vooral in oppervlaktewater welke onder invloed staat van effluent van rioolwaterzuiveringsinstallaties en oppervlakte afstroming van landbouwgrond. . Het is belangrijk om het lot van EDC's te onderzoeken gedurende BF. Op laboratorium-schaal uitgevoerdkolomonderzoek en potjesproeven gaven de primaire mechanismen van EDC's (oestrogeen verbindingen) en brachten de factoren in kaart welke de verwijdering van oestrogeen verbindingen bepalen. Biotische en abiotische experimenten werden toegepast met behulp van potjesproeven om de rol van de microbiële activiteit in de verwijdering van oestrogeen verbindingen te onderzoeken. Bovendien werden de potjesproeven uitgevoerd onder verschillende redox-omstandigheden om het effect van verschillende redox-omstandigheden op de oestrogeen verwijdering te onderzoeken. Op basis van de resultaten kan worden geconcludeerd dat adsorptie en biologische afbraak beide belangrijke verwijdringsmechanismen zijn, waarbij adsorptie het primaire mechanisme bleek te zijn. 17-17-estradiol en ethinylestradiol werden verwijderd voor 99% en 96%, respectievelijk, tijdens de potjesproeven. De factoren gebruikt in dit onderzoek bleken niet van invloed op de verwijdering van 17-estradiol. Echter, 17-ethinylestradiol verwijdering varieerde van 64% tot 87% tijdens kolomonderzoek, welke klaargemaakt waren voor verschillende mate van biodegradatie.

Rol van de biologische afbraak tijdens oeverfiltratie

Natuurlijke zuiveringssystemen zoals BF staan bekend als een effectieve barrière in de meervoudige barrière benadering voor de afvlakking en verwijdering van organische microverontreinigingen. In deze studie werd de rol van de biologische afbraak van geselecteerde PhACs tijdens bodempassage onderzocht. Potjesproeven werden   eerst uitgevoerd om de verwijdering van de 13 geselecteerde PhACs uit verschillende waterbronnen te onderzoeken, om zo de ivloed te zien van verschillende bronnen van biologisch afbreekbaar organisch materiaal. Kolom experimenten werden uitgevoerd om vervolgens onderscheid te kunnen maken tussen de biologische afbraak en sorptie op de verwijdering van geselecteerde PhACs. Geselecteerde neutrale PhACs (phenacetine, paracetamol en cafeïne) en zure PhACs (ibuprofen, fenoprofen, bezafibraat en naproxen) hadden een verwijderingsrendemente van meer dan 87% met verschillende watermatrices tijdens de potjesproeven (verblijftijd: 60 dagen). Verwijderingsefficiëntie van de geselecteerde zure PhACs (ibuprofen, fenoprofen, bezafibraat, ketoprofen en naproxen) was minder dan 35% onder abiotische condities. Dit werd toegeschreven aan sorptie onder abiotische omstandigheden, welke warden gecreeerd door het toedoenen van een biocide (20 mM van natriumazide), die de microbiële activiteit / biologische afbraak onderdrukt. Echter, onder biotische omstandigheden was het verwijderingspercentage van deze zure PhACs verbindingen meer dan 78%, voornamelijk toe te schrijven aan biologische afbraak. Bovendien was de gemiddelde efficiëntie van de verwijdering van hydrofiele (polaire) neutrale PhACs met een lage octanol / water coëfficiënt (log Kow <2) (paracetamol, pentoxifylline, phenacetine en cafeïne) laag (<12%) onder abiotische condities. Echter, onder biotische omstandigheden was de verwijdering van geselecteerde neutrale PhACs meer dan 91%. In tegenstelling hiertot had carbamazepine een persistent gedrag in zowel potjesproeven als tijdens kolomonderzoek. In het algemeen heeft deze studie aangetoond dat de biologische afbraak een belangrijk mechanisme wasn voor het verwijderen van PhACs tijdens bodempassage.

De verwijdering van organische microverontreinigingen uit drinkwaterbronnen tijdens oeverfiltratie en kunstmatige aanvulling van grondwater

Natuurlijke zuiveringssystemen, zoals BF en AR (kunstmatige aanvulling) zijn robuuste barrieres voor veel OMPs en vormen een goedkoop alternatief ten opzichte van geavanceerde technieken voor de productie van drinkwater. Deze studie analyseert een uitgebreide database van Omps op BF en AR locaties in de buurt van Lake Tegel in Berlijn (Duitsland). De focus van de studie was op de afleiding van correlaties tussen het verwijderingspercentages van OMPs en de belangrijkste factoren die de prestaties van BF en AR bepalen. Op de BF locatie staan ondiepe peilbuizen in oxische zones dicht bij de bron Lake Tegel, gevolgd door langdurige zuurstofloze omstandigheden in diepe peilbuizen op grotere afstand van de bron, richting productie. Op de AR locatie golden oxische omstandigheden vanaf de infiltratieplas tot aan de winputten. Bij de BF lacatie zorgen lange verblijftijdenvan 4,5 maandvoor afvlakking van de temperatuur tussen zomer en winter. De temperatuurschommelingen waren groter bij de AR locatie, als gevolg van kortere verblijfstijden. Bij de BF locatie waren de diepe peilbuizen en de winputten onder invloed van grondwater en oud oeverfiltraat (tot een paar jaar oud). Opmenging met andere bonnen moet dus meegeonem worden bij het vaststellen van de verwijderingscapaciteit van OMP's tijdens vodempassage op deze locatie. Principal component analyzes (PCA) werd gebruikt om de correlaties tussen de OMP verwijdering en hydrogeochemische omstandigheden van de beide locaties te onderzoeken. Voor de BF locatie was de belangrijkste component-1 (PC1) redoxcondities en de hieropvolgende belangrijkste component (PC2) het afbraak potentieel (bv. het totale organische koolstof en opgelost organisch koolstof) samen met het calciumcarbonaat oplosbaarheidspotentieel (Ca2 + en HCO3-). Deze twee PC's namen 55% van de variantie voor hun rekening, bij de BF locatie. Bij de AR locatie bleken door de PCA analyse redoxcondities (PC1) en potentiële degradatie met de temperatuur (PC2) als belangrijkste componenten, die een totale variantie van 56% bevat.

Kader voor de beoordeling van organische microverontreinigingen tijdens kunstmatige oppervlakte infiltratie

Kunstmatige oppervlakte infiltratie (MAR, bijv. BF en AR) is een betrouwbaar en bewezen proces, waarin de kwaliteit van het water tijdens bodempassage door verschillende fysische, biologische en chemische mechanismen wordt verbeterd. Zoals hierboven vermeld, kan MAR mogelijk worden opgenomen in een meervoudigebarrière systeem voor de verwijdering van OMPs tijdens drinkwater behandeling en het hergebruik van afvalwater. Echter, er is wel een behoefde aan de ontwikkling van een beoordelingsmethodiek. In deze studie werden richtlijnen ontwikkeld voor de verschillende klassen van organische microverontreinigingen, waaronder de verwijderingsefficiëntie van deze verbindingen kan worden bepaald als functie van de reistijden en afstanden. Richtlijnen zijn opgenomen in Microsoft Excel-spreadsheets en een eenvoudige tool is ontwikkeld om de verwijdering van verschillende klassen van Omps in te schatten. Multiple lineaire regressie analyse van de gegevens verkregen uit de literatuur toonden aan dat de reistijd een van de belangrijkste parameters is in het schatten van de prestaties van een systeem voor PhAC verwijdering tijdens MAR. Bovendien is een kwantitatieve structuur activiteit-relatie (QSAR) gebaseerd model voorgesteld om de verwijdering van OmMPs te voorspellen. De QSAR benadering is vooral handig voor verbindingen met weinig informatie over hun gedrag tijdens bodempassage.

Praktische implicaties van de bevindingen en aanbevelingen voor verder onderzoek

Op basis van de bevindingen van deze studie kan worden geconcludeerd dat BF een effectieve barrière is, in de meervoudige barrière benadering voor het verwijderen van organische microverontreinigingen tijdens drinkwaterproductie. De verwijdering van OMPs tijdens BF kan worden gemaximaliseerd door een goed ontwerp van de winputten, rekening houdend met de waterkwaliteit van de bron en de lokale hydrogeologische omstandigheden. De studie laat zien dat de meeste organische microverontreinigingen kunnen worden verwijderd gedurende een oeverfiltratie stap, zij het in verschillende mate. Meer dan 50% van bulk organische stof wordt verwijderd tijdens de eerste paar meter. Echter, de studie liet ook zien dat voor de in deze studie gekozen PhACs een minimale afstand van 55 meter nodig is voor de verwezenlijking van ten minste 50% verwijdering. Met uitzondering van de Rontgencontrastmiddelen welke een langere verblijftijd lieten zien, hebben de meeste stoffen na verblijftijden van minstens 20 dagen een minimale verwijdering van 50%. Het is ook belangrijk om genoeg verblijftijd te hebben (bijvoorbeeld 60 dagen) tijdens BF om biologisch stabiel filtraat te verkrijgen. In het algemeen zijn oxische omstandigheden gevolgd door zuurstofloze omstandigheden tijdens bodempassage effectief voor het verwijderen van redox-gevoelige organische microverontreinigingen. Een belangrijke conclusie van deze studie is dat enkel MAR, niet geschikt is voor het verwijderen van alle organische microverontreinigingen. Het is dan ook belangrijk om een juiste nabehandeling van MAR te kiezen , om deverwijdering van organische microverontreinigingen te maximaliseren. BF gevolgd door nanofiltratie is een effectieve combinatie.

Alhoewel de mechanismen biodegradatie, sorptie en afvlakking een verwijdering van OMPs bereiken, is de beste benadering om de lozing van deze stiffen vanuit huishoudns en afvalwaterzuiveringen te minimaliseren. .

De ontwikkelde richtlijnen voor de groepen van organische microverontreinigingen kunnen verder worden verbeterd om hun betrouwbaarheid te verhogen, door meer literatuurbronnen te gebruiken. gedetaileerde studies naar de mogelijke directe opname van PhACs door micro-organismen als koolstofbron is nodig, omdat de PhACs niet altijd getransformeerd worden door het co-metabolisme. Verder onderzoek is noodzakelijk om het lot van organische microverontreinigingen tijdens bodempassage te onderzoeken met behulp van verschillende soorten bodems. Meer onderzoek moet worden uitgevoerd op de combinatie van MAR met andere geavanceerde waterzuivering processen (bijvoorbeeld, geavanceerde oxidatie en ionenwisselaars). Dit zou het drinkwaterbedrijven helpen de beste combinatie van zuiveringstechnieken te kiezen voor de verwijdering van organische microverontreinigingen.

LIST OF PUBLICATIONS

International referred journals

Maeng, S.K., Sharma, S.K., Amy, G.L., Magic-Knezev, A., 2008. Fate of effluent organic matter (EfOM) and natural organic matter (NOM) through riverbank filtration. Water Science & Technology, 57(12), 1999–2007.

Baghoth, S.A., Maeng, S.K., Salinas Rodríguez, S.G., Ronteltap, M., Sharma S.K., Kennedy M., Amy, G.L., 2008. An urban water cycle perspective of natural organic matter (NOM): NOM in drinking water, wastewater effluent, storm water, and seawater, Water Science & Technology: Water Supply, 6(8), 701-707.

Maeng, S.K., Ameda, E.A., Sharma, S.K., Grützmacher, G., Amy, G.L., 2010. Organic micropollutant removal from wastewater effluent-impacted drinking water sources during bank filtration and artificial recharge. Water Research, 44 (11), 4003-4014.

Maeng, S.K. Sharma, S.K. and Amy G.L., 2010. Modelling of removal of wastewater-derived organic micropollutants during managed aquifer recharge and recovery, Water Science and Technology, Accepted.

Yangali-Quintanilla, V., Maeng, S.K., Fujioka, T., Kennedy, M., Amy, G.L., 2010. Proposing nanofiltration as acceptable barrier for organic contaminants in water reuse, Journal of Membrane Science, 362, 334-345.

Book Chapters

Maeng, S.K., Sharma, S.K., Amy G.L., 2010. Framework for assessment of organic micropollutant (OMP) removals during managed aquifer recharge and recovery (MAR): In "Riverbank filtration for Water Security in Desert Countries", C. Ray and M. Shamrukh (eds), NATO Science for Peace and Security Series, Springer, Dordrecht, The Netherlands, (In Press).

Sharma S.K., Baghoth, S.A., Maeng, S.K., Salinas Rodríguez, S.G., Amy, G.L, 2011. Chapter 3. Natural Organic Matter: Characterization Profiling as a Basis for Treatment Process Selection and Performance Monitoring. In "Handbook on Particle Separation Processes", A. van Nieuwenhuijzen and J. van der Graaf (eds.), IWA Publications (In Press).

Sharma, S.K., Maeng, S.K., Nam, S., Amy, G.L., 2011. Chapter 68. Characterization Tools for Differentiating NOM from EfOM. In "Treatise on Water Science", Volume 3: Aquatic Chemistry and Microbiology, Elsevier Publications (In Press).

Publications in preparation

Maeng, S.K., Sharma, S.K, Lekkerkerker, K., Amy, G.L., Occurrence and fate of bulk organic matter and pharmaceutically active compounds in managed aquifer recharge, Submitted to Water Research.

Maeng, S. K., Abel, C.D.H., Sharma, S.K., Park, N.S., A., Amy, G.L., Effects of microbial activity and dissolved organic matter removal on geosmin and 2-methylisoborneol during managed aquifer recharge, Submitted to Water Science and Technology.

Maeng, S. K., Abel, C.D.H., Sharma, S.K., Magic-Knezev, A., Amy, G.L., Role of biodegradation in the transformation of dissolved organic matter and removal of pharmaceutically active compounds during managed aquifer recharge: batch and column studies, In preparation.

Maeng, S.K., Sharma, S.K., Magic-Knezev, A., Amy, G.L., Fate of pharmaceutically active compounds in wastewater-derived surface water during managed aquifer recharge, In preparation.

Conferences proceedings

Maeng, S.K., Sharma, S.K., Magic-Knezev, A., Amy, G.L., 2008. Characterization of bulk organic matter upon soil column passage to simulate the impact of wastewater effluent during riverbank filtration, Netherland Scientific Symposium, Soil and Water, 9-10, June, 2008, Zeist, The Netherlands.

Amy, G.L., Maeng, S.K., Jekel, M., Ernst, M., Villacorte, L.O., Yangali Quintanilla, V., Kim, T.U., Reemtsma, T., 2008. Advanced water/wastewater treatment process selection for organic micropollutant removal: a quantitative structure-activity relationship (QSAR) approach. In: Singapore International Water Week, 23-27, June, 2008, Singapore.

Maeng, S.K., Ameda, E.A., Sharma, S.K., Grützmacher, G., Amy, G.L., 2009. Riverbank filtration and artificial recharge and recovery for organic micropollutants removal - NASARI, Korean Society of Environmental Engineers Biannual Conference, 30 April - 1 May, 2009, Changwon, South Korea.

Amy, G.L., Ameda, E.A., Sharma, S.K. Maeng, S.K., Grutzmacher, G., 2009. Bank Filtration of Wastewater-Impacted Drinking Water Sources: A Robust and Effective Barrier for Organic Micropollutant Elimination in Indirect Potable Reuse 6th IWA Leading-Edge Conference on Water and Wastewater Technologies Leading Edge 2009, 23-25, June, 2009, Singapore.

Maeng, S.K. Abel, C.D.H., Sharma, S.K., Amy G.L., 2009. Impact of Biodegradability of Natural Organic Matter and Redox Conditions on Removal of Pharmaceutically Active Compounds during Riverbank Filtration, High Quality Drinking Water Conference 2009, 9-10, June, 2009, Delft, the Netherlands.

Maeng, S. K., Sharma, S.K., Amy, G.L., 2009. Framework for assessment of organic micropollutant removal during soil/aquifer-based natural treatment processes, NATO workshop 2009, 24-27, October, 2009, Luxor, Egypt.

Maeng, S.K., Abel, C.D.H., Sharma, S.K., Amy, G.L., 2009. Effect of biodegradable organic matter and microbial activity on removal of geosmin and 2-MIB during riverbank filtration, IWA Benelux Regional Young Water Professionals Conference, 30 September - 2 October, 2009, Eindhoven, The Netherlands.

Maeng, S. K. Sharma, S.K., Amy, G.L., 2010. Modelling of removal of wastewater-derived organic micropollutants during managed aquifer recharge, Proceedings of the IWA World Water Congress and Exhibition, 19-24, September, 2010, Montreal, Canada.

CURRICULUM VITAE

Sung Kyu (Andrew) Maeng was born in Seoul, South Korea on 5 January 1972. After finishing secondary school from Hoosac School, New York, USA, he started B.S. in Environmental Engineering at Rensselaer Polytechnic Institute (RPI), Troy, New York, USA and graduated in May, 1995. From 1995 to 1997, he carried out research at Georgia Institute of Technology, Atlanta, Georgia, USA for his M.S. thesis, entitled "Effect of a silver-bearing photoprocessing wastewater and silver compounds on biological treatment process", under guidance of Prof. Spyros Pavlostathis. He started his career at Korea Institute of Science and Technology (KIST), Seoul, South Korea in 1999. In 2006, he joined Ph.D. research at UNESCO-IHE/Delft University of Technology on "Multiple objective treatment aspects of bank filtration". Currently, he is a senior researcher at KIST, Seoul, South Korea.